PERSONAL CAREGIVER HANDBOOK

GLORIA LOPEZ

Order this book online at www.trafford.com
or email orders@trafford.com

Most Trafford titles are also available at major online book retailers.

Print information available on the last page.

ISBN: 978-1-4907-8072-6 (sc)
ISBN: 978-1-4907-8073-3 (e)

Library of Congress Control Number: 2017901590

Trafford rev. 08/21/2017

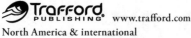 www.trafford.com

North America & international
toll-free: 1 888 232 4444 (USA & Canada)
fax: 812 355 4082

Contents

Special Thanks

To my son, Michael, and the many families who have a family member requiring the assistance of a caregiver and understand the importance of documenting daily information.

To caregivers who have been helpful, understanding, and providing the care needed to ensure a continuum of health and by keeping the family, client, and the medical team informed of what has occurred.

To Debra Butler for her continued support and offering recommendations through her personal experiences of the importance of documentation.

About the Author

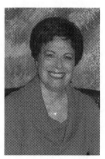 For over forty-two years, Gloria A. Lopez has worked with children with disabilities and their families and with adults who were diagnosed with medical conditions later in life.

A mother of three children, her son was born with a disability—spina bifida. Her experiences led her to design books that offer an individual self-empowerment by taking a more active role in their medical care through documentation.

As a parent of a young adult with multiple anomalies since birth, the challenges presented by the professionals involved and the many changes in the health condition as well as the transitional evolution to an adult provided the purpose for the development of this book and the hope that if a transfer of care was necessary, there would be a minimal break in the daily care with the medical information provided. It has ensured the continuity of the health of her son. The record keeping from a caregiver has provided invaluable information when a medical situation arose, being available to share the information with the medical team assisting with the diagnosis.

Ms. Lopez believes that documenting your medical history and daily care will help prevent and minimize medical errors and assist the medical team. She is a speaker and an advocate on the purpose of documentation and has authored *Personal Medical Journal, My Personal Medical Journal, Personal Medical Pocket Journal, Personal Caregiver Handbook,* and *Personal Care Handbook.*

Personal Caregiver Handbook

Gloria A. Lopez

The *Personal Caregiver Handbook* is designed to assist the caregiver to understand the medical needs of an individual or client and the importance of documenting daily information. An individual or whom ever has the responsibility of providing and overseeing the care of an individual requiring a caregiver will generally prepare the personalized handbook; such as a sibling caring for a family member, a spouse, a parent, an individual, or a conservator. The information charted provides the opportunity to have the most pertinent personal daily information in the event a medical situation occurs, and recognizes the valuable component the caregiver offers.

> *I found as a parent of a young adult with multiple anomalies since birth, the challenges presented by the professionals involved, and the many changes in the health condition as well as the transitional evolution to an adult provided the purpose for the development of this book. It ensured the continuum of health of my son while utilizing a caregiver and was a work in progress over several years. The record keeping from a caregiver has provided invaluable information when a medical situation arose. I could share the information with the medical team, assisting with a diagnosis.*

It's important to understand that even though you will find many forms included and it may appear overwhelming take one step at a time. Start with the most important area selecting one form and then adding another as needed. I have provided many ideas to help you with what may be needed, and you will find that you may require additional information from time to time.

We frequently do not realize the detail of care that is required to ensure the tasks, comfort, safety, and continuum of care. When you consider the following examples, you may find it very surprising:

1. The number of times you need to remind the individual of a task, i.e. you ask the person to drink something, etc.
2. How long does it take to do each task?
3. Accompanying to appointments.
   a. Preparation, driving, rescheduling an appointment, etc.
4. Grocery shopping and errands
   a. Shopping lists, grocery store, pharmacy, retail stores, etc.
5. Laundry instructions
   a. Wash, dry, put away, laundry supplies replenished.

      b.   How to use the washer and dryer.

      c.   Amount of a laundry product and what to use for specific items.

6. Medication

      a.   Ordering, organizing the medication tray, distributing, etc.

7. Medical supplies

      a.   Ordering, organizing, what is their responsibility, etc.

8. Preparing a meal

      a.   Menus, preparing meals, clean up, and kitchen kept in a clean environment.

9. Trip planning

      a.   Packing, ensuring all medication and supplies required are included for length of the trip, and any additional equipment.

Provided for you are forms to use as guidelines. You can customize them to your needs with the digital copy that is available online at www.LCPBooks.com or by contacting our office at info@lcpbooks.com. Make multiple copies and have the caregiver complete the daily forms you require, such as the Daily Vital Record Keeping, Monitor Log, Caregiver Daily Checklist, etc.

When customizing your handbook, it is important to understand you will be dealing with your raw emotions that can be exhausting. As Ms. Lopez was informed by her physician years ago, *"Take your emotions and attitude and put them in a can with a lid,"* you can bring out your emotions later. The importance is to ensure the care you require is recorded and getting the needed service and funding available. Be honest with each item you document to assist the social service or agency you are working with to better understand the care needed.

Be clear with your social worker when seeking a funding program for assistance that you are providing the clarity needed to assist the continuum of health for the individual who requires a caregiver. The area you live may have some strict guidelines that could involve child or adult protective services. If you consider this as an option, you may want to discuss it with your physician first to understand what it provides you that includes any limitations, legal issues, and advantages and disadvantages for your particular situation. Thereby, unless you believe a protective service is necessary, you may want to be prepared with a note from your physician stating what they recommend as they know the family/individuals care dynamics to ensure there is not a misunderstanding of what you are requesting for the service or funding program you are seeking.

Please remember to *customize* the material to meet your specific needs.

➢ The caregiver is here to assist in the daily care.

➢ It will be important to be honest and provide essential information so the caregiver will be able to handle the care appropriately while maintaining a continuum of health.

➢ The documented information is important to assist any caregiver of what has previously occurred and what is expected to best perform their daily duties.

➢ Daily documentation provides the primary caregiver and the individual with information needed when a medical situation or emergency occurs.

➢ Keep all data and information in lay terms, not in professional terminology that will make it difficult to read and follow, so anyone can understand.

➢ The information supplied should be kept in strict confidence for the individual and whoever they want to read the handbook. The caregiver should be informed *not* to share any personal information outside of the home.

➢ There will be information within this book that you may not need, and that will be to your discretion.

➢ Feel free to add data to best assist you and the caregiver.

It is recommended to have a medical health summary and a portable health journal, such as the *Personal Medical Journal*, to assist the caregiver if there is an emergency or when they accompany their client to various medical appointments.

There is the option to have the caregiver fill in some of the included forms on the computer or complete manually and maintain in the daily binder.

When using the *Personal Caregiver Handbook*, preprinted forms customize it to fit your needs and be sure to make extra copies. ALWAYS keep one as a master copy to have available for future usage.

To begin, purchase the following and any other items that would provide you the tools necessary to keep the information in an easy-to-use binder:

1. One three-ring binder that is a minimum three-to-four-inches capacity from your local supermarket, office supply store, or pharmacy
   a. To hold your forms and other information
2. Dividers tabs for various forms and care instructions
   a. Divide into easy-to-use sections for your convenience.
3. Annual monthly calendar divider
   a. Add the set to the binder as suggested in the sections forms list.

4. Plastic 8.5 x 11 business card holders
   a. This makes it easy to reference specific vendors, service providers, medical team, and any other resource that is valuable for the caregiver in the event of an emergency, pharmacy or supply order, etc.
5. The forms that are preprinted are *samples*. You can customize any form shown within this handbook to meet your individual needs by purchasing a disc that includes all forms. The disc is available through the Life Cycles Publishing office.
   a. Included in the disc is a table of contents. You can use these titles to make it easy for labeling each section to correspond with the preprinted forms or adding a section title with your individual form.
   b. You will notice that individually, the forms contain daily charted information that should be taken to a doctor or emergency visit, such as Daily Vitals Record Keeping, Intake Log, plus any additional pertinent information you have added. Sections are explained further in the sections forms list on the following pages.
6. Use a three-hole punch for the forms to add to the binder.
7. Plastic holders or pocket dividers and store behind the annual calendar section to hold any extra form copies

You may want to check with a legal advisor to discuss which legal documents to consider for your loved one. Inquire how to protect their assets, which include the advantages and the disadvantages. Understand their importance or why they are needed, the procedures required, the financial costs, and any other questions or concerns so you can be informed of the options available. The following are some documents to consider:

1. Emancipated Child vs. Unemancipated Child. A child can be discharged or remain dependent regarding the care from their parent. Discuss how this affects the individual when they are over the age of eighteen (18) years and the various funding and service programs available.
2. Special Needs Trust. An irrevocable trust in which the disabled beneficiary's assets are protected to remain eligible to the various funding and services available.
3. Conservatorship. A guardian or a protector is appointed to manage the financial and/or daily life of another because of a physical or mental limitation or old age. If you have a special needs trust, discuss the appropriate conservatorship to consider one or both of the following:
   a. If only for *medical*. Generally, if you manage the special needs trust, this may be all you will need but discuss this with your legal advisor.

b. If a *financial* is needed. Be sure to discuss the meaning and the procedure when needing to obtain funds.

4. Advanced Health Directive. A document that makes provisions for health care decisions in the event the person becomes incompetent to make such a decision.

5. Power of Attorney. Written authorization to represent or act on another's behalf to make decisions if the signer is unable to make such decisions.

6. Any other legal venue in your state or country to consider to protect your loved one.

This is especially important if your loved one is over the age of eighteen (18) years. It allows anyone to share or discuss information with you from one or more of the following services: a health-care service provider, the medical team, during a doctor's visit, while in the hospital, or with various social service agencies.

It is important to contact your current program providers of any changes, especially should there be a change in the primary caregiver or a move to a new location outside the area you are receiving services. Be sure to ask what the procedure is and the appropriate paperwork or documents required to ensure there is a continuum of service. This will assist to make an easier transition and especially helpful for the new person who is handling all the paperwork.

Therefore, it is important to keep all your files in a location that is easy to access for anyone who may need to take over the responsibility of caring for your loved one or yourself.

Consider this *Personal Caregiver Handbook* as a tool to assist you. There will no longer be a need to memorize every detail regarding the medical history, helping to eliminate the redundancy of information. The health-care professional is pleased to know that you have your information organized. This will help contribute to optimum care.

Remember, *Personal Caregiver Handbook* preprinted forms have a copyright, and unauthorized distribution is illegal.

Congratulations! You now have the comfort of accuracy and assistance with the daily personal care and monitoring needed.

The Caregiver

Blessed are those individuals who assist another with their daily care. A person filled with the compassion and love that they want to enhance an individual who has a disability or limitation is exceptional. It takes a strong spirit to be able to maintain the patience needed, guidance to improve an individual's daily life, and the appropriate care that is involved.

I want to thank all those caregivers who have given of themselves offering a caring hand, a warming smile, and the knowledge they have blessed an individual and their family. Assisting an individual who benefits from the care offered provides a sense of strength and empowerment and lets another person know someone cares.

The family is so thankful for your tenderness and loving ways, so they can be at peace knowing they have assistance, a peace of mind, and that their loved one is being cared for appropriately.

The *Personal Caregiver Handbook* was designed to assist an individual who needs assistance and the primary caregiver when a caregiver is hired. It provides the guidelines and tools for documentation and the information a caregiver will need to provide the appropriate care and understand what is requested of them.

It will take time to organize your personalized handbook. Start by taking those sections that are primary at first and build as the need arises, knowing you have the information needed. By setting up your own handbook, it can assist you when sharing what you have designed with the various service agencies you may utilize to obtain additional services. This can provide additional clarity as to extent of care needed.

You can contact the office of Life Cycles Publishing at info@LCPBooks.com to obtain a digital copy of the forms for you to customize for your needs, remembering all forms are copyrighted and protected.

By organizing your *Personal Caregiver Handbook*, you will be able to have a peace of mind that you have established a central place for the caregiver to be able to refer to for their guidance in the daily care needed.

Forms List

The caregiver needs to understand the importance of all the forms to be completed daily. There is a disc available through the Life Cycles Publishing office that has separate fill-in forms you can customize to meet your needs available.

1. **Address A to Z**
   a. Contact information regarding all medical, service agencies, suppliers, etc.
   b. Include a business card holder: Ask each individual who assists you for their business card.
   Note: You may want to put a note on the card, add the date, and something to remind you of the purpose of the provider or addressee.

2. **Alerts and Concerns Log**
   a. It is important to list any medical, physical, or emotional areas of concern that require attention.
   b. Keep updated as situations arise.

3. **Allergy List**
   a. This is important to keep up to date and include all allergies, such as foods, medication, herbal supplements, environmental, etc.

4. **Caregiver Daily Checklist** (also included in the Caregiver Hiring Packet)
   a. It is extremely important to keep detailed documentation of all tasks performed for the person with special needs.
   b. This will assist with funding and program services. Various service programs will use these documents to determine eligibility, and the accumulation of per-minute tasks can assist to increase the financial assistance.
   c. Start by making a list:
   - Each time you need to do any task, no matter how simple, document it on an individual line, stating how often it is required and how long it takes. The actual time required to perform the various daily tasks will surprise you.
   - There will be times when an illness or surgery recovery will require more care; document these tasks on this form since it can be a reoccurring situation. If there is a time when a task is not required, mark it as not needed.

- Depending on the medical condition, you may want to make the list based on the worst day, which requires the most care as it may be difficult to determine when it may different. You can always make a change to your original form daily. The service provider and social worker will need to know this information to better assess the needs they are providing to assist you.

- There may be some items that a hired caregiver would not be authorized to do depending on the provider service you are using. Request the limitations in writing as you may want to look for a service that will best fit your needs.

d. The caregiver will need to check off their tasks daily and place in the appropriate month with the most current date on top.

5. Caregiver Hiring Packet

This area is meant to assist the individual who will require a caregiver to assist with daily home care and the primary caregiver who is seeking assistance and provides information on how to hire a caregiver, an interview sheet, and instructions once you have hired a caregiver or service:

a. Caregiver Agreement

b. Caregiver Daily Checklist (located in section 4)

c. Caregiver Employment Application

d. Caregiver Guidelines

e. Caregiver Hire Guidelines

f. Caregiver Interview Checklist

g. Caregiver Interview Evaluation

h. Caregiver Interview Guidelines

i. Caregiver Interview Questionnaire

j. Caregiver Job Description

6. Caregiver Sign-In Log

a. The caregiver should sign in and out daily, especially when there is a rotation of caregivers.

b. The areas filled in will help in the future to know who worked on a shift and their contact information should the need arise. Be cautious if you are writing any notes on the caregiver that another individual could read and possibly misinterpret.

c. Keep additional blank copies available in the back of the binder.

7. **Chart Notes**

   a. Use this form to leave a note regarding an occurrence or medical concern or as a daily update.

   b. It will alert any other caregiver on a situation that has occurred or requires monitoring.

   c. This allows the caregiver to make a daily note of what occurred during the day.

8. **Community Transportation**

   a. Guidelines to assist with mobility instructions for any form of community transportation: bus, train, rapid transit system, etc.

   b. Feel free to customize it to meet your needs.

9. **Daily Vital Record Keeping**

   a. This is *very important* to chart several times daily.

   b. This will be a *critical* form to *take* to a doctor's visit or if an emergency arises.

      • If needed, have the nurse make a copy of the form for their file.

   c. Feel free to customize it to meet your needs.

10. **Emergency Contact Information**

    a. The individual or the primary caregiver needs to complete this information.

    b. Make a copy and post it on a cabinet or refrigerator for easy access.

11. **Equipment Maintenance**

    a. Sample form showing how to use, care needed, and precautions for any equipment that is utilized.

    b. Separate fill-in section of this form for you to customize to meet your needs.

    c. Be sure to add all equipment and the specific needs for its care.

12. **Intake Log**

    a. Helps monitor all food and liquid intake.

13. **Laundry**

    a. The caregiver will be handling the laundry and you want to ensure they do it to your specifications.

    b. It will be important to have some instructions for them to follow.

    c. Don't assume everyone washes or dry's clothes the same as you and will know how to use Your machines.

14. Meal Suggestions

    a.   Provides helpful meal suggestions.

    b.   If the individual has sensitive food allergies, take a copy when admitted into the hospital to assist the dietician with suggestions.

15. Medical Concerns Checklist

    a.   When an illness or medical condition occurs, this section describes how the caregiver can best assist the individual. It is also helpful for the medical team when an emergency arises.

    b.   It will be important that all information is thoroughly documented and kept up to date.

    c.   Separate fill-in section of this form for you to customize to meet your needs.

16. Medical Occurrence Log

    a.   This form is used when a medical condition occurs to keep everyone abreast of a situation.

    b.   To prevent future confusion, use one form per type of medical situation. This will maintain an independent frequency log of reoccurring events, such as urinary tract infections (UTIs), seizures, falls, etc.

    c.   Keep additional copies available in the back of the binder.

17. Medication Daily Schedule and Medication Chart Schedule

    a.   This is *very important* to keep up to date, especially when medication needs to be distributed by the caregiver.

    b.   Keep a copy with the medication bottles.

18. Monitoring Log

    a.   This is an optional form as you can keep similar information in the Daily Vital Record Keeping Log to be used as needed.

19. Personal Bag Organization

    a.   Quick reference for any items needed when leaving the home.

    b.   Separate fill-in section of this form for you to customize to meet your needs.

20. Personal Medical Summary

Summarize all past and current health information.

    a.   If you are unable to recall the exact date, use the approximate year.

b. Surgeries and procedures (If you do not remember the exact name, give a brief explanation.)

c. Complete as much history as you can remember and feel free to include all pertinent information that will be helpful during an emergency or medical treatment.

d. State if there is a particular medical condition that needs to be considered for future reference. Something that occurred even years prior could have an impact on a situation that is occurring today, and the medical team will need to know to better assist you with a diagnosis and recovery.

e. Make copies of the summary and keep a current master for your files.

21. Personal Supplies

a. List all supplies and reorder information used, such as incontinence care and medical supplier contact information, etc. State if it is on automatic reorder, frequency, and when to place the order as needed.

b. Make an up-to-date Personal Supplies reorder form available for reordering with the suppliers' contact information.

Binder Organization Suggestion

This provides a suggestion on how to organize your binder for easy caregiver access. *Remember*, this is your binder, and it is important to have what you believe to be the pertinent information a caregiver may need to provide the services that you are requesting.

A. **Purchased annual calendar monthly divider**
   1. Use this to collect the daily log sheets and all information by month.
   2. Caregiver should keep each log or notes used for daily charting in chorological order with the current date on top.
   3. This will allow the primary caregiver easy access to the daily information.
   4. Take the pertinent forms when seeing a medical professional or if an emergency arises to share what has occurred over several days or weeks and return them to the binder after the visit.
   5. At the end of the year, remove the monthly information and place it in a file for future reference.

B. **First section:** Contains the pertinent daily information
   1. Caregiver Sign-In/Out Log
   2. Emergency Contact Information
   3. Meal Suggestions
   4. Allergy List
   5. Medication Daily Schedule
   6. Alerts and Concerns Log
   7. Medical Concerns Checklist
   8. Medical Occurrence Log
   9. Equipment Maintenance
   10. Community Transportation
   11. Personal Supplies List
   12. Personal Bag Organization
   13. Address A to Z

C. **Annual monthly calendar dividers**
   1. This is for the forms that you want to monitor daily.
   2. It provides easy access and organization in the event you need to take a form that has the history to a medical appointment.

D. **Section to hold all your forms:** Have several blank copies available for a minimum of one to two weeks.

You can put each form set in a three-hole ring plastic holder or with pockets for easy access.

1. Caregiver Daily Checklist

2. Daily Vital Record Keeping

3. Monitoring Log—Blood Pressure, Glucose, Other

4. Intake Log

5. Medical Occurrence Log

6. Personal Supplies fax/call reorder form. Create a list of the product numbers, information, and amount to recorder. The caregiver can simply check off which supplies are needed.

7. Chart Notes

8. Any other forms you have designed to best assist you

9. Blank note paper for notes and daily instructions as needed

1
Address A to Z

Maintaining a list of all your service providers, medical team, medical suppliers, etc., allows for an easier access when they need to be contacted. This allows you to build your resources that can be helpful today and in the future.

Include a business card holder that is available to purchase through your local office supply store. Ask each individual or business who assists you for their business card. By adding a note on the card—the date you met, location, and anything that will remind you of the purpose of the provider or addressee—it makes it easier to remember the individual or the company.

As you will notice, there are categories listed on the top of the address form in case you may want to categorize the various contacts by their specialty for an easy access.

You can always add A to Z dividers or regular blank dividers that you can obtain at your local office supply store to make your personal address resource section.

Always keep in mind *this is your Personal Caregiver Handbook* to assist you and the caregivers who assist you.

Address A to Z   ❑ Doctor • ❑ Hospital • ❑ Service/Agency • ❑ Therapist • ❑ Other

Name_____

Phone_____ Other_____

Specialty_____

Hospital/Clinic_____

Address_____ Ste/Room_____

City_____ ST_____ Zip_____

E-mail Address_____

Note_____

◆

Name_____

Phone_____ Other_____

Specialty_____

Hospital/Clinic_____

Address_____ Ste/Room_____

City_____ ST_____ Zip_____

E-mail Address_____

Note_____

◆

Name_____

Phone_____ Other_____

Specialty_____

Hospital/Clinic_____

Address_____ Ste/Room_____

City_____ ST_____ Zip_____

E-mail Address_____

Note_____

◆

Name_____

Phone_____ Other_____

Specialty_____

Hospital/Clinic_____

Address_____ Ste/Room_____

City_____ ST_____ Zip_____

E-mail Address_____

Note_____

2
Alerts and Concerns Log

It is important to list any medical, physical, or emotional areas of concern that require attention. It will assist the caregiver of a medical condition that needs to be monitored. Document when it occurs on the Medical Occurrence Log and the Chart Notes as well as to notify the primary caregiver and possibly, the physician.

This can be used when there is an emergency. Take a copy with you when you see a medical professional and give to the emergency team. This can help assist to better establish the cause of a medical situation quicker or to eliminate a possible procedure, especially in an emergency.

Be sure to keep the information up to date as each situation arises.

Alerts and Concerns Log

It is important to list any medical, physical, or emotional areas of concern that require attention.

Maintain a log for easy recall and review.

	Date	Condition	Concern
1.			
2.			
3.			
4.			
5.			
6.			
7.			
8.			
9.			
10.			
11.			
12.			
13.			
14.			
15.			
16.			
17.			
18.			
19.			
20.			

3

Allergy List

It is important for you to keep this up to date and include all allergies, especially if there are any that are life-threatening. State what the medical condition is as well as any remedy instructions, medications to administer immediately, what to look for, and if an ambulance is needed. It is recommended to keep a list in the wallet for easy access.

- Foods
- Medication
- Herbal supplements
- Environmental, etc.

Food Allergy Card

Have a Food Allergy Card to show to the restaurant server who can show it to the manager and the cooks of any food allergies so they can help ensure your safety and for you to have a nice experience in the restaurant. We have them available upon request, or you can easily purchase a business card format from your local office supply store and print it in your language. I recommend using the back of the card for another commonly used language in your area, for example, one side in English and the other in Spanish. Then you can have it laminated at your local business office center, such as Kinkos, Staples, etc.

Ms. Lopez has found this to be a lifesaver as there have been many times when upon inquiry, the server would think they do not use an allergy product in their restaurant. Later, when the card is shown to the chef or the manager, they would find out that it is the product that was actually used in the food preparation. There should be careful consideration or directions for a type of menu item so that it is safe to eat as well as in the kitchen to ensure that there is no cross-contamination of the food preparation area with the kitchen tools used or the need to alter the recipe. When you are in a banquet setting, give your card to the hostess so they can have the banquet manager check for you. Do not be fooled that because it is an exclusive setting or high-quality facility, they always use top-end products, and a preservative is not used if this is your allergy. It is to *save your life* and to enjoy your time with your family and friends or just a time of solitude. Better safe than sorry or having to go to a hospital.

Example: You can state whatever you are comfortable with, but remember, this is to help keep you safe and possibly save your life depending on the allergic reaction. It is important to have your name included as either the manager or chef may want to meet you to discuss food options.

MY NAME (for the manager to find you)   **FOOD ALLERGIES**
 	
Life-Threatening (*examples of what to state*)
   • Dairy, gluten,
   • Nuts, shellfish, etc.
Additional Food Sensitivities:
   • List any foods here individually.

On the back, you could repeat this in Spanish. If you do not know how to spell a word, you can ask someone who speaks the language; or in your grocery store, you could look for food labels on items where they are sometimes in English and Spanish so you can have a reference. Remember, depending on the country, the food item could be spelled differently, so you may need to be alert for this.

Allergy List

❑ **MEDICATION** ❖ ❑ **FOOD** ❖ ❑ **OTHER**

Keep each category on a separate page.

DATE	CAUSE OF ALLERGY State medication or food	REACTION Explain symptoms i.e., rash, anaphylaxis, etc.	REMEDY Counteractive action i.e., specific medication
1.			
2.			
3.			
4.			
5.			
6.			
7.			
8.			
9.			
10.			
11.			
12.			
13.			
14.			
15.			
16.			
17.			
18.			
19.			
20.			

4
Caregiver Daily Checklist

It is extremely important to keep detailed documentation of all tasks needed for daily care. Many funding sources and social service programs qualify their services by the time and task needed for the individual's needs. Different tasks performed by a caregiver may appear simple and commonsense, but to a person being considered to assist with caregiving, it may not be a task normally done as each individual requires different considerations to maintain a continuity of health and care. This sample is meant to assist you in considering areas that you will want a caregiver to do. You may want a caregiver to use it daily; therefore, be sure to make copies so they can document that they have done each task as requested.

    *Be sure to customize for the individual's needs.

    *Also, keep an updated copy in the *Personal Care Handbook* and *Caregiver Handbook*.

Start by making a list:

Each time you need to do any task, no matter how simple, document it on an individual line, stating how often it is required and how long it takes. The actual time required to perform the various daily tasks will surprise you.

There will be times when an illness or surgery recovery will require more care; document these tasks on the Caregiver Daily Checklist since it can be a reoccurring situation. If there is a time when a task is not required, mark it as not needed.

There may be some items that a hired caregiver would not be authorized to do depending on the provider service you are using. Request the limitations in writing as you may want to look for a service that will best fit your needs.

Be sure to share this with any service or funding provider to ensure you are receiving the optimum services needed.

Caregiver Daily Checklist

*This is a sample. Be sure to customize for the individual's needs.

*Also, keep an updated copy in both the *Personal Care Handbook* and *Caregiver Handbook*.

Name_____Date_____

It is important to offer assistance when applicable.

Please check each area after you have completed the task.

_____TRANSPORT SERVICE to appointments if needed. Check the schedule for future appointments; some transport services require twenty-four to forty-eight hours prior notification.

- Be sure to make the necessary transportation arrangements for all appointments.
- If you use a transport service, they will need *name, address, phone,* and *appointment time.*
- See the Community Transport section for more instructions.

I. SHOWER - PERSONAL GROOMING SKILLS. Be sure to use gloves and ask what assistance is needed.

_____ 1. Leaves alone if requested. Stay close and within earshot, however, in the event you are needed.

_____ 2. Transferring to shower or tub?
- If using a shower chair, assist with legs and feet protection and placement.
- Placing feet on a stool in the shower helps with stability and prevents hot water burns.

_____ 3. Turn on water and check water temperature.
- Legs and feet burns can occur from water being too hot.

_____ 4. Assist to wash any areas difficult to reach as needed.

_____ 5. Shower complete; check to ensure the water is turned off.

_____ 6. Check frequently for decubitus sores.

_____   a. After the shower, it is an easy time to do a quick visual body check for skin breakdowns, such as an open sore, redness, and skin discoloration on the back area, buttock, elbows, legs, feet, and toes.

_____   b. Clean and dry between the toes. Mention if the toenails need trimming, or you notice a sore or any other condition that may need attention.

_____ 7. Continue to ask if any assistance is needed.

_____ 8. Leave alone to complete grooming skills if requested, staying close and within ear shot in the event you are needed.

_____ 9. Caregiver needs to do a visual check, remind, and/or assist:

    a. Skin check

    b. Teeth cleaning

    c. Ears cleaning

    d. Application of deodorant

    e. Application of cologne, perfume

    f. Fingernails trimming, if applicable

    g. Shaving

Very Important: Ensure that briefs and pants are pulled up correctly so that it minimizes any bulk pressure against the skin when sitting. This can be a cause for a decubitus and needs to be monitored for correct placement of undergarment and pants.

_____ 10. Mention if you observe an odor. Locate source.

    a. Urine: If there is a strong odor or discoloration, it could mean the possibility of a urinary tract infection (UTI). Contact the primary caregiver and/or the doctor on file.

    b. Incontinence: The individual may need a change, shower, or bath.

    c. Sore: Needs immediate attention and to notify the primary caregiver and/or the doctor.

    d. Other_____

_____ 11. Notify primary caregiver of any supplies needed.

II.   **PREPARATION FOR DAY.** Use gloves as needed.

_____ 1. Make bed: Check sheets and change if applicable. Put dirty sheets in the laundry room.

_____ 2. Clean and straighten up bedroom. Vacuum and dust.

_____ 3. Check the daily schedule of activities and pack the travel or backpack with appropriately medical supplies when leaving the home for any period.

_____ 4. Assist with **daily medications** and what medications may need to be taken while on an outing.

    • See: Personal Bag Organization

    • If a prescription *refill* is needed, notify primary caregiver and/or individual.

    • See Medication Daily Schedule and Chart.

_____ 5. Prepare and assist with *breakfast* and *lunch*.

_____ 6. Prepare and assist with *dinner* when needed. If leaving the food for later, cover and place in refrigerator.

_____ 7. **REMINDERS:** Observe the individual and assist to prevent falls and regarding the following:

_____   a. Monitor the intake of medications

_____   b. Monitor the Daily Vitals Checklist and Chart.

_____   c. Chart the fluid intake if needed.

_____   d. Use the Chart Notes section, charting daily regarding the day's events, care, and any occurrence, such as a fall or any other situation, especially noting any problems or concerns, to include grocery or supplies that will be needed.

_____   e. Periodic weight shifting when sitting for long periods to help prevent decubitus ulcers. The physician or therapists may recommend the frequency.

         • Weight shifts every_____minutes when sitting for long periods.

_____   f. Observe and assist with incontinence care if applicable. If you smell or notice soiled clothing, a change is needed.

_____   g. Assist in the daily schedule for appointments and activities.

_____   h. Prepare for appointments and activities that will require assistance.

_____   i. If transportation is needed, contact a service and provide the information needed (see the Community Transport section for more instructions).

_____ 8. **CUSHION:** Use a waterproof pad to prevent from being soiled if applicable.

_____   a. If used with a seating device, wheelchair, etc., check the following:

         1. Is the cushion or cover soiled or smelly?

         2. Do not wash the cushion in a washing machine as it will deteriorate the foam material unless otherwise directed.

         3. Wash only the removable cover.

         4. Follow the Equipment Maintenance section to know what you need to do.

_____   b. Depending on its type, a cushion may require specific care. The individual or the primary caregiver will direct you or review the Equipment Maintenance section for more information.

_____   c. For back cushion, check if in proper placement if applicable.

_____   d. Furniture cushion may need a waterproof pad.

_____ 9. **WHEELCHAIR.** Check if a repair is needed. Contact the primary caregiver.

_____   a. If the tire air pressure is low, assist with pumping tires or take to nearest bike shop.

_____   b. Check if brakes and all parts are working correctly, that is, footrest, armrest, seat belts, etc.

_____ c. Power chair batteries will need to be charged daily and checked periodically.

_____ 10. **HOUSEKEEPING: bedroom, bathroom, kitchen, general living areas**

_____ a. In the bathroom, completely clean the shower, bathtub, toilet, sinks, and floor daily.

_____ b. With laundry, wash, dry, fold, and put away all laundry. Follow the instructions provided regarding the type of soap to use and all laundry products as well as drying instructions.

- Be sure to notify the individual or primary caregiver when laundry products need to be purchased.

_____ c. Clean kitchen. Wash, dry, and put away the dishes, leaving the kitchen neat and in order.

_____ d. Vacuum and mop floors as needed.

_____ e. Dust the surface areas as directed and needed.

_____ f. Water plants as directed and needed.

_____ g. Make a list of any grocery, cleaning, and laundry items needed from the store.

III. **OTHER: Please list all that you want to be handled.**

1. _____ (Prompt to drink to keep hydrated, e.g.)
2. _____ (Frequency to change incontinence care, e.g.)
3. _____ _____
4. _____ _____
5. _____ _____
6. _____ _____
7. _____ _____
8. _____ _____
9. _____ _____
10. _____ _____

5

Caregiver Hiring Packet

This area is meant for assisting the individual who will require a caregiver to assist with daily home care and the primary caregiver who is seeking assistance. Each area provides information from how to hire a caregiver, an interview sheet, to instructions once you have hired a caregiver or service.

Caregiver Agreement

This will provide a clear understanding of a written agreement with your caregiver. It will be important to make the appropriate changes to meet your needs.

Caregiver Daily Checklist. This is located in section 4.

This is important to establish what task is needed in detail for the daily care. Include this form with your hiring packet so the prospective caregiver understands what will be expected of their duties.

Caregiver Employment Application

This is to be completed by the applicant. This will help during the interview to better understand the individual you are hiring. You may want to take a photo with your camera or cell phone for your file. It is important to know your local and state regulations of what you can ask so an applicant does not feel they have been discriminated against.

Caregiver Guidelines

This provides the caregiver guidelines or expectations. Be sure to customize it to ensure clarity of understanding between you and the caregiver of their responsibilities and expectations.

Caregiver Hire Guidelines

The supplied forms within each area give you example guidelines to put in your binder. It will be important for you to customize each area to ensure that your needs are met by adding pertinent information as this is *your* personalized handbook.

Caregiver Interview Checklist

This schedule provides you with guidelines when setting up for an interview.

Caregiver Interview Evaluation

This helps in the applicant elimination process when you have interviewed several applicants. Many of the questions during an interview can reflect a gut feeling about someone. You may want to get a picture to add to your file to help what the applicant looked like; you can use your cell phone for this.

Caregiver Interview Guidelines

This offers information and assistance designed to provide some tools when you need to hire a new caregiver for your loved one or yourself.

Caregiver Interview Questionnaire

This is to be completed by the applicant so you can see if they meet your needs.

Caregiver Job Description

It is important to have a job description to provide clarity on the responsibilities needed, salary, and hours required. Provided is a sample to assist you. You can use some of it and add information or create your own; the choice is yours as this is meant as an example, and your specific needs must be stated to ensure that the applicant understands what is requested of their service. It's important to understand that you are not allowed by law to discriminate on race, sex, age, sexual orientation, religion, marital/family status, arrest history, financial status, or disability. It is important to state if you only want a male or female because of the personal privacy required for care. Here is an example; the individual requiring care is a female, and a female caregiver is needed, etc.

Caregiver Agreement

This will provide a clear understanding of a written agreement with your caregiver. Make the appropriate changes.

DATE_____

Employee _____ SS No. _____

Address _____ City _____

Zip _____ Driver's License No. _____

Phone _____ Other _____

In case of emergency: Name _____ Relationship _____

Phone _____ Or _____

("I" in this document reflects the employee.)

1. I agree to work and perform the duties described on the job description and the daily program schedules discussed as well as any other duties applicable.

2. I accept the salary of $_____per hour and agree to work_____hours daily.

    ❏ Monday ❏ Tuesday ❏ Wednesday ❏ Thursday ❏ Friday ❏ Saturday ❏ Sunday
    ❏ Holidays

3. Because of the nature of my position, I want to state any medical or physical restriction(s) that could create a problem or limitation to fulfill some of the requested daily duties.

    Do you want to explain briefly?   ❏ YES ❏ NO

    _____

    _____

    _____

4. I will not expect pay for any nonworking days to include sick days, holidays, and personal days.

5. I understand that I will receive a schedule and sufficient notice not less than twenty-four (24) hours if I will not be needed unless an emergency or medical situation has occurred.

6. I have answered all the questions in the interview with accuracy and honesty.

7. I do not expect to receive medical insurance.

8. I understand I will be responsible for any tax reporting necessary.

9. I understand I will be paid by ❏ Personal or a ❏ Service_____

❑ Other_____

ACCEPTED: _____   Date _____
             Employee Signature

             _____   Date _____
             ❑ Primary caregiver or ❑ Individual requiring the caregiver

Caregiver Employment Application

We are an "equal opportunity employer." Submission of application does not guarantee employment. ***Please complete and return.***

Personal Information

Date_____

Name_____Social Security No._____
Address_____
City_____State_____Zip_____
Phone_____Cell_____
E-mail_____

Employment Desired

Position_____Date you can start_____
Salary Desired _____
Are you employed? ❑ No ❑ Yes, explain _____

Education History

High School_____Year graduated_____
College or trade school_____Year graduated_____
Field of interest ❑ Nursing _____❑ LVN ❑ NA ❑ OT ❑ PT
❑ Other _____
Graduation/Certification_____

General Information

Special training_____
_____
_____

Prior Employment Okay to contact for reference_____

1. Name _____Phone_____

    Date started_____Ended_____

    Reason for leaving_____

    Please explain briefly job duties_____

    _____

2. Name _____Phone_____

    Date started_____Ended_____

    Reason for leaving_____

    Please explain briefly job duties_____

    _____

Caregiver Guidelines

This provides the caregiver guidelines of expectations. You can customize it to ensure clarity. A caregiver professional should add value to the daily life of the individual. Consider your position as an important aspect for the safety of the person you care for as it is an honor to care for another person.

Remember, you are not babysitting but assisting an individual who has special needs with their daily care.

Ways to protect yourself:

- Take a notepad with you when you go to work to ensure you have paper to write down all information needed. Remember to leave it as you do not need to take it with you since it is personal information. Ask your client where you can leave your notes for future reference.
- Documenting your work will assist you to keep the family informed.
- Accurate documentation of your participation in their daily care adds value to your skills, giving you the opportunity to show the individual and the family you care for their health and safety.
- Should a situation arise, you will know through your documentation you did what was needed.
- Always state any area of care that makes you uncomfortable immediately. This will protect you and allows the individual or primary caregiver to make any necessary changes.

Ask specific information for the following:

1. Individual's name and pertinent information
    a. What is the medical condition or disability, that is, cognitive issues, stroke victim, dementia, other?
    b. Do you distribute medications, and what is the frequency?
    c. Are there any mobility limitations? Are there any specific instructions?
        i. Do they need assistance in walking, for example, with a cane, walker, etc.?
        ii. Do they need assistance in transfers from a bed, chair, commodes, etc.?
        iii. In what other areas does the individual needs to be kept safe or monitored?
    d. Are there any specific medical concerns that you need to monitor or watch for?
    e. If you need to assist with a medical procedure, what do you do, that is, vitals, insulin monitoring, shots, other?

2. Address and cross street (In the event of an emergency, we can get nervous, and having this information is important.)

3. House phone number

4. Contact information of primary caregiver

5. If an emergency occurs, who do you contact?

6. Are there any pets in the home, and do you have any responsibility to them? If you are uncomfortable with this, please state your concerns immediately.

7. What are your duties and responsibilities?

    a. Food preparation

        i. Are there any restrictions or allergies?

        ii. Are there any prepared meals to warm?

        iii. If you are asked to cook, are there any meal suggestions?

    b. Liquid intake: in drinking, do you need to prompt to drink?

    c. Hygiene care: What is involved? How much do you need to do?

        i. Do you assist with showers/baths? Personal grooming? Be sure to find out explicitly in this area so it is not uncomfortable for you or the individual.

        ii. How do you handle an individual's personal needs?

        iii. This is time to check if there are any open sores or red pressure marks.

        iv. Change the briefs (diaper) to ensure they are properly clean.

    d. Changing the bed linen and towels?

    e. Washing laundry, drying, and folding and where to put them in the appropriate cupboard or shelf. As well, what laundry products do they want to be used for the different type of washing loads and drying instructions?

    f. How do you use the various appliances, such as the washing machine and dryer?

    g. Vacuum the bedroom and living area?

    h. Dusting?

    i. Cleaning bathroom?

    j. Taking garbage out and the location of the outside garbage container?

    k. Any other chores requested?

8. Medical situation has occurred, or you notice a problem. What do you do?

    a. Be sure you give your report to the primary caregiver.

    b. Document what happened.

        i. Who do you contact, and where are the phone numbers?

        ii. Be sure to include in your documentation who you reported the situation to and include the time and date.

        iii. Sign your name as this will be needed for future reference.

    c. If 911 is called, are the following information available?

        i. A specific medical facility to go to

        ii. Doctor's name and phone number

        iii. Insurance information

        iv. All medical card numbers and their location to include state/federal agency qualifying programs (e.g. Medi-Cal for California)

        v. Medical history summary

        vi. Medication list or the medication in their Rx containers

        vii. All food and medication allergies

        viii. Is there a personal medical history journal to document what has occurred when going to the hospital or medical appointment?

    d. Have you documented accurately what you did to assist before and after the emergency team arrived?

BE SURE TO ASK IF THERE IS ANYTHING YOU SHOULD BE AWARE OF!

Caregiver Hire Guidelines

The supplied forms within each area give you example guidelines to put in your binder. It will be important for you to customize each area to ensure your needs are met by adding pertinent information as this is your personalized handbook.

1. **Caregiver interview checklist**. This will provide guidelines when preparing for an interview.

   a. For the initial interview meeting, *do not meet at home.* Meet at a fast-food restaurant, coffee shop, or some other neutral location.

   b. Review the questions and add important areas that you want to ensure are covered.

   c. You may want to get a picture of the person to add to your file; you can use your cell phone to help remind you of what the applicant looked like.

   d. *Do not hire until* you have a personal interview and have gone through all the background and reference checks.

   e. If the person *does not* sound like they will work out, say so and thank them for the call or interview.

   f. You may really like the person, but they may be apprehensive about the care. Do not try to make the person do anything they are not comfortable doing. You have the option to limit the chores they will do, but remember, someone will have to do it!

   g. Be sure to add a separate sheet or notebook with additional questions you may have.

2. **Caregiver job description.**

   a. This requires your individualized comments.

   b. Have this with you when you interview and show the person you are interviewing so they can see what is expected of their service.

3. **Caregiver employment application and questionnaire.**

   a. Because you will require specific care needs, you may want to modify this form.

   b. This needs to be completed by the prospective caregiver. Have them fill it in prior to interviewing or visiting with them so you can reference it when talking to them.

4. **Caregiver guidelines**. This should be given to the prospective caregiver to provide guidelines for questions and expectations.

5. **Caregiver Daily Checklist**. Be sure to make the appropriate changes (located in section 4).

   a. Make a *detailed list* of your expectations of care to ensure that all needs are met.

b. Every time you do even a simple task, add it to your list, that is, get drinks, simple reminders, etc.

c. The caregiver is hired to assist the individual with their care and assistance with their needs in the home, *not* the entire household chores unless you make other arrangements.

d. Caregiver household chores list: clean the bathroom and kitchen daily, laundry, vacuum, mop, dust, cook, shop, etc., *not* babysit, watch TV, or personal reading.

e. You *may* want to hire another person to clean the home weekly or biweekly depending on your needs. The caregiver could do the surface cleaning and another person or service to handle the more intense cleaning.

6. **Caregiver interview evaluation**

    a. This is for your reference only and best for your records as it is not intended to be shared with the applicant.

    b. Areas are in general topics for reminders.

    c. Add additional specific topics and information that fit your needs.

    d. The responses to the questions during an interview can give you a gut feeling about someone. Once you become more familiar with the person and with the background check, you will be able to make a more informed decision regarding hiring.

    e. This helps in the applicant elimination process when you have interviewed several applicants.

Important Safeguards to Consider

Insurance. When hiring a caregiver, be sure to contact your personal insurance agent to ensure you are protected in the event of a claim regarding the following and ask the type of coverage it offers:

a. It is recommended to add a workers' compensation insurance policy to your homeowner's policy. The premium is generally extremely low, and it gives you important protection. If you are working with a health provider service, they should have a policy so be sure to request a copy or certificate of insurance so you know you are protected. Do not assume because they have a business that they have the appropriate insurance that protects the employee so always ask.

b. Mention to your personal automobile agent that the hired caregiver may use your vehicle for errands to ensure you have the appropriate coverage; or the hired caregiver may use their personal vehicle, and you want to ensure if they are driving your loved one to appointments, errands, or anything, they have the appropriate insurance coverage. Ask for an insurance certificate, and to be sure the coverage is appropriate, you can have your personal agent review it.

Discrimination. Be careful not to discriminate because of religion, race, or sex. Be open to the individual who has the appropriate experience to handle your needs safely. However, it is okay to state upfront that the person who requires the care may be more comfortable with a specific person, such as a male or a female.

    a.   A small-structured female may not be able to handle an adult male when transferring or when handling incontinence issues.

    b.   A female may be very uncomfortable with a male caregiver.

State and local required documents. Contact the following local offices for the required documents when hiring an employee.

    a.   Labor Commissioner Office

    b.   Employment Development Department

Be sure to ask if there are other offices to locate and obtain the contact information as well as any areas and helpful suggestions to be considered.

Health service provider. This is an important service as they are experienced and can handle all the background checks needed and more. There is an additional charge but well worth the additional comfort of knowing you have done your best when hiring someone to care for your loved one and who is coming into your home.

    a.   Fingerprinting

    b.   Credit report checks

    c.   Felony or misdemeanors

    d.   Motor vehicle records (important if they are going to drive for you)

    e.   Drug testing

    f.   Reference checks

    g.   Ask what other services are offered.

Payroll. This can get difficult with the payroll taxes if you are personally handling and not using a health service provider. If personally handling, you may want to contact a payroll service to assist you as you are required to pay and file the state and federal taxes and appropriate reporting.

Caregiver personnel file. Keep a copy of all the hiring and payroll information for *each* caregiver in their individual personnel file.

Appliance and equipment

a. Have instructions for each household appliance used, such as the washing machine (how to separate clothes, types of laundry products used, etc.), clothes dryers (i.e., clean lint filter), coffee maker, and others.

b. If there is a particular equipment they need to check or use, it will be important to have instructions. You can use the Equipment Maintenance section to assist you.

Home protection/security

a. Put a lock on any door the caregiver will not need to enter.

b. Protect all valuables and medications and place in a secured location that will not be accessible.

c. Contact a local security monitoring service for options and suggestions, and you may want to add cameras. Using these services provides you to go online via your computer and on cell phones to view what is occurring while you are away.

d. You can get a nanny-cam type of camera available online to help monitor what the caregiver is doing when you are not present.

e. Be sure to keep the bills, all receipts, and any personal information in a protected location to help prevent identity theft.

Caregiver Interview Checklist

This checklist provides you with guidelines when setting up for an interview.

Name_____Date_____

Phone ❑ Cell_____❑ Home_____❑ Other_____

E-mail_____

1. Discuss basic chores before meeting. If still interested, then arrange for a meeting.
2. Set up: Date_____ Time_____Location_____
3. Job Description. Have a copy for the prospective caregiver to review and return.
4. Employment Application. Have the interviewee complete and review each area with them during the interview.
5. Availability.
   a. Days: ❑ Monday ❑ Tuesday ❑ Wednesday ❑ Thursday ❑ Friday
   Attending College_____

         ❑ Full time   ❑ Part time

         ❑ Availability   Days _____ Hours _____

         ❑ Units_____Major_____

   b. Employed Where _____

         ❑ Full time   ❑ Part time

         ❑ Availability   Days_____Hours_____

         ❑ Can I contact them_____ If yes, ask for the supervisor name and phone number.

         _____

6. Caregiver Questionnaire. For you to use to ask questions for the interview.
7. Caregiver Daily Checklist. Discuss duties explicitly.
8. Show *Personal Caregiver Handbook* with the different sections.
   a. Explain medical history summary to understand the medical condition.
   b. Emergencies or medical attention. *What to look for and whom to contact.*
   c. Equipment. Be sure to mention any equipment and supplies used. See the Equipment Maintenance section.
9. Ask if he/she is interested in the job. This is also a time for you to decide if you want to hire this person.
10. Inform the person if you work with a health service provider and that they will handle all background, credit, fingerprinting, and reference checks. Ask if this is agreeable; if not, it can be a clue not to hire.
11. Discuss when you will get back to them regarding the hiring decision, time, and date_____
12. Notify the health service provider with the name and phone number of the prospective caregiver to begin the background, drug, and credit check.

13. Once you have decided to hire, give the prospective caregiver the number to the health service provider you have selected to begin the process.

14. Salary $_____. Have a range. Start low, but it must be at least minimum wage. However, it is best to have it *slightly* higher than minimum wage depending on what would be required.

15. Be sure if you will be using a funding source to cover the salary. Explain what they will need to do to register with the service provider.

    • Ensure you understand the hourly wages provided by the service provider and the prospective employee accepts the wages.
    • You have an option to add another source or personal funds to provide a higher wage.
    • It will be important to discuss the various salary funding options and ask if they accept.

16. Hours. List days and times required.

17. Employment duration. Length of time available for employment_____

18. Any existing medical conditions with limitations that would prevent doing what is required (i.e., back problems, disability, walking or lifting limitations, etc.). You can decide if this person is appropriate for your needs if a disability will prevent them from fulfilling what is needed. Be careful as you are not to ask and they are not required by law to disclose, only if offer the information voluntarily or you observe a situation.

Use this section to add any questions you may have.

_____ 19. _____
_____ 20. _____
_____ 21. _____
_____ 22. _____
_____ 23. _____
_____ 24. _____
_____ 25. _____
_____ 26. _____
_____ 27. _____
_____ 28. _____
_____ 29. _____
_____ 30. _____
_____ 31. _____
_____ 32. _____
_____ 33. _____
_____ 34. _____
_____ 35. _____
_____ 36. _____
_____ 37. _____
_____ 38. _____
_____ 39. _____

Caregiver Interview Evaluation

A.   The following is for *your reference only*. Areas are in general topics for reminders. Add additional specific topics and information that fit your needs.

B.   This helps in the applicant elimination process when you have interviewed several applicants.

C.   Many of the questions during an interview can reflect a gut feeling about someone.

D.   Once you become more familiar with the person and with the background check, you will be able to make a more informed hiring decision.

E.   You may want to get a picture to add to your file to help remind you of what the applicant looked like; you can use your cell phone for this.

NAME_____**Date**_____

Health Service Provider. Contact for the background check and start date of employment.

     Name_____

     Contact_____Phone_____

     Address_____

     E-mail_____

_____1. **Prospective Caregiver APPEARS.** You can review their personal appearance and vehicle to see if it is kept clean and neat. Watch for any other clue that will help you see how they will care for your needs.

❑ YES ❑ NO a.   Dependable.

❑ YES ❑ NO b.   Honest.

❑ YES ❑ NO c.   Able to work independently.

❑ YES ❑ NO d.   Social lifestyles compatible.

❑ YES ❑ NO e.   Would you be comfortable with this person in your home when you are not present?

❑ YES ❑ NO f.   Does he/she appear neat?

_____2. **Personality**

❑ YES ❑ NO a.   Friendly.

❑ YES ❑ NO b.   Appears to get along with others

❑ YES ❑ NO c.   Enjoys working with families with special needs

_____3.**Hours**

❑ YES ❑ NO a. Willing to work flexible hours and different shifts. ❑ A.M. ❑ Afternoon

❑ P.M. ❑ Evenings

❑ YES ❑ NO b. Attends college.

❑ YES ❑ NO   If yes, are the hours flexible enough to accommodate both schedules?

❑ YES ❑ NO c. Do they have another job?

❑ YES ❑ NO   If yes, are the hours flexible enough to accommodate both schedules?

❑ YES ❑ NO d. Flexible. Able to assist with your time management as needed and willing to adjust to change regarding working hours.

_____4. **Duties**

❑ YES ❑ NO a. Willing to do cleaning, cooking, and domestic chores either assigned or as needed?

    i.   Reviewed the Job Description.

    ii. Reviewed the Caregiver Daily Checklist that includes household chores of what will be expected.

❑ YES ❑ NO b. Accepts the personal care duties and responsibilities (i.e., issues of bowel, bladder, vomiting, etc.) If not, in what areas?_____

_____5. **Medical Knowledge**

❑ YES ❑ NO a. Has had medical training? If yes, explain._____

❑ YES ❑ NO b. Licensed? If yes, explain._____

❑ YES ❑ NO c. Has the basic knowledge of what to do in an emergency.

❑ YES ❑ NO d. CPR/first aid certified?

❑ YES ❑ NO   If no, willing to take a class? Note: Offered through the American Red Cross or online.

_____6. **References**. Note: If the reference is family or a friend, you will only receive positive comments.

❑ YES ❑ NO a. Willing to work with a health service provider who will do a complete background check, fingerprinting, and drug testing that will include all references verified?

❑ YES ❑ NO b. Reports from health service provider are in good standing. If not, you can ask the person what occurred; and if they explain, then you have the opportunity to make the final decision to hire.

_____7. **Drives**

❑ YES ❑ NO a. Have the health service provider check the motor vehicle report (MVR)?

❑ YES ❑ NO b. Do they have a vehicle available to handle errands and appointments, such as going to the pharmacy, taking a specimen to a laboratory, or going to the grocery store or to another location?

❑ YES ❑ NO c. If yes, are they willing to use their vehicle?

❑ YES ❑ NO d. Proof of automobile insurance limits. Ask for a copy of their insurance declaration page to see what type of coverage limits they have.

Note: Add to your personal insurance the nonowned vehicle coverage to ensure that if they are doing errands, you are covered under your auto policy. Check with your insurance agent to ensure that you have the insurance protection.

❑ YES ❑ NO e. Travel. If willing to accompany on a trip for any period.

Note: This would be used on an individual basis or until sometime in the future as an option once you have decided if you can trust this individual.

_____8. **Salary**

❑ YES ❑ NO a. Has accepted the salary range offered $_____per hour? It is best to have an hourly rate.

❑ YES ❑ NO b. Willing to accept payment from other funding agencies?

_____9. **Medical Conditions**. A health service provider can ask some of the delicate questions.

❑ YES ❑ NO Do they have any medical condition that would limit them from doing what is requested? You do have the right to ask this question.

Discuss this area with your health service provider to ensure they give you the legal guidelines to follow in your state or local area, or they can ask the questions and report the responses to you. Make an additional list to ensure that your needs are met.

Here are a few areas to consider: Ask your service provider if they can ask the personal health questions and any suggestions or recommendations.

❑ YES ❑ NO a. Lifting. Any weight restrictions?
If yes, get an explanation.

❑ YES ❑ NO b. Mobility issues?
What type of mobility issues?

❑ YES ❑ NO c. Disabled?
What is the disability?

iii. It also gives you time, ninety (90) days, to see if the person you hired is appropriate for your needs.

iv. Negotiate with the health service provider on their hourly salary under their contract. Remember that you must pay the minimum wage and ask the length of time needed to be kept under their contract until you can have the person under your direct payroll. This would mean you would be completely responsible for the person's payroll, taxes, and workers' compensation insurance.

v. Generally, a caregiver does not expect health benefits and vacation or sick leave pay as this can be an option should you want to offer.

vi. You can start the person at a lower hourly wage and increase once they have completed their ninety-day probation and under your payroll versus the health service provider.

vii. You may want to consider a payroll service that will handle all the taxes and filings required.

It is recommended utilizing the Web to search for information to assist you. Here are a few references:

1. www.AARP.org. You may need to be creative to find some of your answers, but I have found they have good information that can be used for any age regarding caregivers and finding a facility to assist you with a loved one.

2. www.CareInHomes.com. They have a very informative interactive website.

3. Check the search engines with the topic on the type of disability, caregiver, home facilities, etc.

Caregiver Interview Questionnaire

Applicant (Please complete and return to the person you are interviewing with.)

DATE_____

NAME_____PHONE_____

E-MAIL_____CELL_____

❑ Male ❑ Female

Field of Interest: ❑ Nursing_____ ❑ LVN ❑ NA ❑ OT ❑ PT

License Type /Specialty

❑ Other_____

1. How many years of education have you completed?_____

2. ❑ YES ❑ NO Are you new to the area? Explain._____

3. What types of work have you done and liked the best?_____

_____

4. ❑ YES ❑ NO Do you have previous experience working with a person with a disability?
    Explain._____

5. What are your feelings toward disabilities?_____

6. How do you deal with boredom and stress?_____

7. ❑ YES ❑ NO Will you be able to drive or accompany to appointments when needed?

8. ❑ YES ❑ NO Are you comfortable using your vehicle for errands and/or doctor appointments?
    ❑ YES ❑ NO Do you have car insurance?

    You will be requested to provide a copy of the declaration sheet from your auto policy
    that shows the coverage limits if you will be driving your car for errands and doctor
    appointments and a copy of your current motor vehicle record.

9. ❑ YES ❑ NO This position may require lifting or positioning. Your response is optional only
    if you want to disclose. Do you have any physical or emotional limitations that would
    limit your job?
    If you are comfortable to explain further, please use the back side of this paper.

10. ❑ YES ❑ NO Are you comfortable with lifting and assisting with transfers.
    Explain any limitations._____

11. ❑ YES ❑ NO Can you work independently?

12. ❑ YES ❑ NO Do you mind working with nudity that goes along with personal care?
    Explain any limitations._____

13. ❑ YES ❑ NO Will you do laundry—wash, dry, fold, and put away?

14. ❑ YES ❑ NO Will you do food preparation and cooking?

15. ❑ YES ❑ NO Will you do household chores? Make bed, clean up bathroom, etc.?

16. ❏ YES ❏ NO Would you be willing to wear the caregiver attire (scrubs or other). *This is an optional personal preference if you want them not to wear their street clothes while at work.*

17. ❏ YES ❏ NO _____

18. ❏ YES ❏ NO _____

19. ❏ YES ❏ NO _____

20. ❏ YES ❏ NO _____

Caregiver Job Description

This is a sample to assist you. You can use some of it and add information or create your own. The choice is yours as this is meant as an example, and your specific needs must be stated to ensure the applicant understands what is requested of their service.

Date_____

DISABILITY _____

CLIENT ❑ Male ❑ Female: ❑ Young ❑ Teenager ❑ 21+ older ❑ _____age if applicable, etc.

DUTIES. *Be sure to personalize anything important for your individual needs.*

1. Review each section of your *Personal Caregiver Handbook* or the *Personal Care Handbook.*

2. Use the Caregiver Daily Checklist to review the daily chores.

   a. Assist with monitoring daily health concerns, guidance, and assistance as needed.

   b. Skin inspection for decubitus, fractures, sores, burns, etc.

   c. Assist with food preparation.

   d. Monitor medication intake and notify primary caregiver if a refill is needed.

   e. Take vitals as needed or required.

   f. When you notice an important medical condition, incident, or illness, notify primary caregiver immediately.

   g. Assist with transfers when applicable.

   h. Assist to reorder medical supplies if applicable.

   i. Light housekeeping. Review Caregiver Daily Checklist.

      i. Assist with keeping bathroom and bedroom clean.

      ii. Make bed and change sheets when applicable.

      iii. Wash, fold, and put laundry away.

      iv. Complete the Caregiver Daily Checklist.

   j. Accompany to doctor appointments or trips (optional).

Provide a resume and a referral list of three (3) past employment references with phone numbers to contact who are not family or friends.

Contact Person (Name)_____**Phone** _____

HOURS   HOURS NEEDED. *Hours may be flexible depending on daily needs.*

Weekly Total_____

Morning_____

Afternoon_____

Evening_____

Other (explain)_____

DAYS NEEDED ❏ Monday ❏ Tuesday ❏ Wednesday ❏ Thursday ❏ Friday ❏ Saturday

                 ❏ Sunday

PAY $_____ ❏ Per Hour ❏ Weekly ❏ Monthly

TIME CARD   Maintain approved hours by ❏ primary caregiver, ❏ case manager or

                 ❏ other_____

BENEFITS   ❏ None ❏ Health ❏ Other *(explain)*_____

We are an equal opportunity employer. Submission of application does not guarantee employment.

6
Caregiver Sign-In Log

1. The caregiver should sign in and out daily, especially when there is a rotation of caregivers.
2. It will help to know who worked on a shift and their contact information should the need arise and if the primary caregiver needs to discuss a situation that occurred during their shift.
3. Keep additional blank copies available in the back of the binder.

Caregiver Sign-In Log

The caregiver needs to sign in and out daily, especially when there is a rotation of caregivers. This will give the primary caregiver the opportunity to contact you should a situation occurred and they need more information.

| | DATE | NAME | TITLE | SERVICE | | TIME | |
				HEALTH-CARE SERVICE PROVIDER	OTHER Explain	IN	OUT
1							
2							
3							
4							
5							
6							
7							
8							
9							
10							
11							
12							
13							
14							

7
Chart Notes

- Use this form to leave a note regarding an occurrence, or medical concern, or as a daily update.
- This will alert the family, primary caregiver, or any other caregiver on a situation that has occurred or requires monitoring.
- This is important to be sure you have protected your client if a fall occurred, or there was something out of the ordinary.
- It is *important* to notify by phone, unless you have been instructed otherwise, the primary caregiver and the physician if a situation occurs that will require any medical attention.

Chart Notes

Use this form to leave a note for the primary caregiver or individual regarding an occurrence or medical concern or as a daily update.

Day_____ **Date**_____ **Time**_____

Person Charting ❑ Caregiver ❑ Nurse ❑ Family ❑ Other_____

Name _____ **Title** _____

Temperature _____ **Blood Pressure** _____

Skin

❑ Good ❑ Discoloration_____ ❑ Wound (Describe below.)

Urine

Color ❑ Clear ❑ Brown/red (bloody) ❑ Odor ❑ Other (Describe below.)

1. Area of Concern   ❑ NONE   ❑ Allergies   ❑ Fractures   ❑ Infection   ❑ Other

_____

_____

Explain/comment _____

_____

_____

_____

_____

_____

2. Area of Concern   ❑ NONE   ❑ Allergies   ❑ Fractures   ❑ Infection   ❑ Other

_____

_____

Explain/comment_____

_____

_____

_____

_____

_____

Signed _____ Notified _____

8

Community Transportation

Guidelines to assist with mobility instructions for any form of community transportation—bus, train, muni, rapid transit system, etc.

It is important to assist the individual with special needs to have the self-confidence so that they can be more mobile with your assistance. Getting a person out of their home environment can provide good self-esteem and the opportunity to be in more social gatherings if at the mall and moving around, to the doctor's visit, store, a church gathering, a movie, school, a time to meet a friend or family, or sports event. It offers a feeling of independence and strength.

There are several options available in an area. Some funding services offer taxi or community transit free passes so be sure to inquire what is available in your area. Ask the distance any one service will provide and if there will be an additional charge.

It is recommended to travel with the individual at first until they are comfortable to be alone. If handling a public transit system, you may want to follow in your vehicle to ensure they get off at the designated destination for a few times until you and they are comfortable to handle it independently.

Be sure to instruct the individual to tell the driver what exit point they will need and to ask where to pick up the return transport vehicle or bus.

Note that some of the paratransit services may not be on your time frame for the pickup or delivery. They may come early or later. So be sure to ask how much time is needed to be ready prior to pickup and the location to meet as well as the approximate time they may be delivered to their destination. If taking any supplies, be sure to have them properly marked in the event they get left on the transport vehicle so the people can notify you they have the bag or item that was left.

Community Transportation

The following are guidelines when assisting an individual with mobility for any form of community transportation—bus, train, muni, rapid transit system, etc.

I. **ROUTING: Instructions**

1. Request local transit schedule - disabled access guide.
   a. Call a local transit service.
   b. Ask for their best route.
   c. Refer to the transportation guide that discusses the schedule, whom to call for information, emergencies, etc.
   d. A community transport service may pick up at the home, take to the destination, and pick up for the return trip.

2. Use index cards.
   a. Using a hole punch, put a hole in upper corner.
   b. Put ring or string through for more than one card.
   c. On each index card, write the following:
   (The following is an example however applicable to any type of transportation system.)

   → *Side 1*
   ✓ **To**_____
   ✓ **From**_____
   ✓ **Destination**_____

   ✓ **Times of departure**_____
                 _____
                 _____

   ✓ **Bus number**_____
   ✓ **Location**_____
   ✓ **Departs / Leaves**_____

   ✓ **Transfers: How many**_____
   ✓ **Bus number**_____
   ✓ **Location**_____
   ✓ **Departs / Leaves**_____

    ✓ **Destination**_____

✱ Be sure to ask the driver for assistance if needed and the location of the pickup area.

   ✱ *Side 2:* On the back of index card, write the return information.

Use the same format as on the front side.

3. Keep information simple; use large writing.

II. BEFORE LEAVING Checklist

1. Take the index card and check time frames.
   a. Call the transportation company for assistance:
      ✓Verify times, current bus line number (such as bus number), route, etc.
      ✓If a lift is required for a wheelchair or any type of assistance needed for individual needs, would they be available?
   b. Allow extra time to get to and from bus stop to the destination.
   c. Keep an ID card in travel pack that has the name, address, bus line needed, phone number, and emergency information.
   d. Fill backpack for travel with supplies and extra clothing.
   e. Take a bottle of water.
   f. Be sure any medications needed during the time away from home are packed.

III. AT BUS STOP
1. **Ramp Safety**
   a. Stay clear from the ramp while in motion.
   b. Wheelchair users generally back onto ramp.
   c. Wheelchair users put brakes on when on the ramp.
   d. Transport services, buses, etc., will not allow a wheelchair without a seat belt and properly working brakes.
2. **On Bus Locking System**
   a. Be sure the chair is secured to the locking system by the transport driver.
   b. Some transport systems also have a seat belt that goes around the wheelchair.
   c. Apply brakes on wheelchair.
3. **Upon Reaching Destination**
   a. Inform the driver of the destination when entering the bus.

    b.   Brace for all stops.

    c.   Inform the driver before reaching the stop.

    d.   Okay to ask for help, directions, etc.

    e.   Ask the driver where the pickup location is for the return trip.

    f.   Check the cross streets needed to reach the return bus location.

IV. CROSSWALK SAFETY

    a.   Use wheelchair ramps.

    b.   Use pedestrian crosswalk buttons if available.

    c.   Carefully check for cars not watching. *Be alert!*

NOTE. When learning to travel independently:

    a.   It is strongly recommended that a caregiver travels with the individual a few times to be sure there is an understanding of the transportation routine.

    b.   When traveling independently, have someone follow in a car to ensure they know their route and get to their destination.

9
Daily Vital Record Keeping

Maintaining a daily vital record is important. By charting daily in the appropriate areas, it provides the individual who requires a caregiver and the primary caregiver valuable information. It can demonstrate a medical concern when the information differentiates from one day to another.

Take it to the doctor's visit to show what the daily charting records show and if further testing or a change in a medication will be needed.

Daily Vital Record Keeping

1. Important to document daily vitals and add notes.
2. Take to the doctor's office.

Date							
Time							
Caregiver Initials							
Blood Pressure Normal ___ / ___							
Pulse Normal ___							
Temperature Normal ___							
Urine							
Odor							
Color							
Skin – Sores, Breakdown							
Location							
Treatment? Explain							
Vomiting No. of times?							
When (i.e., after meal, etc.)							

Sugar Levels Normal ___							
Other							

10
Emergency Contact Information

The individual or the primary caregiver needs to complete this information for quick access of important contact information in the event an emergency occurs.

Place a copy on a cabinet or refrigerator in the kitchen and any other location so it is easily visible and easily accessed.

Emergency Contact Information

Keep this in the caregiver binder and post in an area where it is easily accessible in the event there is an emergency.

Name _____

Address _____

Home Phone _____ Other _____

Nearest intersection _____

Medical Care Service Provider _____ Phone _____

In an Emergency ❑ Medical History Available ❑ Allergies ❑ Medication ❑ Foods ❑ _____

Call 911 and/or ❑ Primary Caregiver _____

Mobile Phone _____ Other _____

Doctor _____ Phone_____

Hospital/Medical Facility _____

Medical Insurance Carrier _____ ID No. _____

Additional Contact:

Name _____

Relationship _____ Phone _____

Additional Important Contacts:

State if family, friend, or other _____

_____

Information to provide the medical team, physician, emergency team, etc.

Take the following:

    ❑ ID and insurance cards (generally found in a wallet unless otherwise directed by primary caregiver)

    ❑ The *Personal Caregiver Handbook* ❑ *Personal Medical Journal*

    ❑ Personal Medical Summary

    ❑ Personal and medical supplies (a medical facility may not have the preferred supplies)

    ❑ All medication bottles and the Medication Daily Schedule

❑ The following individual sheets from the *Personal Caregiver Handbook*:

    ❑ Current Daily Vitals Record Keeping Log ❑ Medical Concerns Checklist

❑ Alerts and Concerns Log

❑ Allergy List

❑ _____

Additional Information ❑ Use the Community Transportation Instruction Section

<u>Transportation</u>

Service _____ Taxi _____

11
Equipment Maintenance

It is important to have information on each equipment used, the vendor's contact number if a repair is necessary, and where specific equipment or supplies can be ordered.

Keeping the information in an area that is simple to access, along with the care instructions, will enable the caregiver to know how to care and whom to contact for repairs or reorder of specific supplies for each piece of equipment that is used.

The attached information will also give you pertinent information on general equipment as to what to consider when purchasing an item and how to use, care for, and precautions for any equipment that is utilized. It will be important to customize it for your needs. There may be areas that you specifically need to have considered or to add a section when reordering or placing an order on an item.

Separating each equipment provides an easy way to find them. Be sure to fill in sections of this form for you to customize to meet your needs.

Equipment Maintenance

Complete this form, customizing it to meet your needs.

Be sure to add all equipment and the specific needs for its care. Be sure to add additional pages with your information on any equipment you may have that is not included.

<u>CONTACT</u>   1. Primary caregiver ❏ See list_____ Phone_____

                    2. Mobility service provider_____ Phone_____

This section includes information on a variety of equipment used and areas to consider regarding the purpose of the equipment, initial ordering, and more on the following:

    I.   Wheelchair

    II.   Cushions, seating and back

    III. Shower chair

    IV. Bags

    V.   Accessories

    VI. Customized vehicles and vans with a lift

    VII. Miscellaneous equipment

    VIII. Additional equipment and information

            a. _____

            b. _____

The individual and the primary caregiver should take time before an item is purchased to understand the purpose and the need for the equipment. It is important to understand the following:

1. Purpose for the equipment

    a.   Always consider the individual needs, activities, and options in style and color.

2. Do you need a prescription?

3. Cost and optional items available

4. Check with insurance or any other service regarding the following:

    a.   Coverage of the purchase and the type of co-pay

    b.   Frequency of replacement (generally, every two to three years or after a surgery)

5. Who handles any repairs?

6. What are the safety considerations?

7. Ask your physician for a mobility service provider referral.

    a.   Equipment orders and repairs are generally through a mobility service provider.

8. When personalizing this section be sure to state the maintenance and where it can be serviced, how to clean, and any pertinent information.

I. **Wheelchair**

1. A prescription from your physician is required for coverage by your insurance.

2. Request reevaluation assessments every two to three years to ensure that the equipment continues to adequately meet the appropriate needs.

3. Work with the mobility specialist to ensure the proper fit, chair height, and balance.

4. Manual, sports, and power chairs. There are various designs to meet your independent style of activity and use. It will be important to inform the mobility specialist on your type of activities to ensure the accuracy of the evaluation.

5. When ordering, *discuss* these important areas with the specialist:

    a. Solid frame versus folding chair. Ask about the pros and cons.

    b. Balance and comfort

    c. Shoulder placement and the center point to the wheel axle. Ensure that the hands maneuver the wheels easily on a manual chair. Correct placement may require various adjustments.

    d. The sitting height, including the cushion of the chair, needs consideration to ensure that a person can fit comfortably under most tables.

    e. Seat belt is an *important safety feature* and required if using public transportation or a transport service while sitting in the chair.

    f. Back of chair height

    g. Sports chairs generally have a lower back height. It is important to ensure safety and security while maintaining balance and comfort.

6. Power chairs require checking the battery daily for charging and maintenance. Use the manufacturer's guidelines for the proper care.

    a. Be sure to ask how to transport. Can it be taken apart easily, and what form of vehicle transportation is recommended?

    b. Will it require a van and a lift purchase? If so, see number VII for guidelines.

7. Seat

    a. The knee edge of the seat length should have a two-finger space from behind the knee to minimize the chance of reduced leg and feet circulation issues as well as proper leg and foot placement.

    b. The seat width needs appropriate space for comfort and stability.

        i. Consider the distance of the arm reach with manual chairs to have proper shoulder extension while wheeling.

    c. The correct angle can provide stability, balance, and comfort. This is important when a chair is ordered.

     i. Too much of a seating angle (aka bucket angle) can cause problems by adding pressure to the blood supply and nerves that can affect balance.

       • A bucket refers to the seat angle between the front and back that can vary by specific degrees.

     ii. Discuss the options and how it will best meet your needs.

     iii. Sports or daily activity may have an effect on the degree angle.

8. Small front-wheel casters: The size and type of wheel can make a difference in maneuverability.

9. Tires

    a. There are several *types* of tires, wheel sizes, and camber angles to consider for maneuverability. Some of the areas to consider are as follows:

     i. Shoulder extension

     ii. Balance

     iii. Height for your leg and feet position and table height

     iv. Many individuals find that having a camber angled allows for easy maneuverability, especially for sports activities.

       • Be sure to watch the camber angled to fit in doorways.

     v. Always ask your mobility specialist for more considerations.

       ➢ Note:

         • Using tube liners will help prevent flat tires or ask your dealer for other alternatives.

         • Tires should be checked frequently by the caregiver to maintain good air pressure.

         • The side of tire will tell you the appropriate air pressure.

         • You can purchase tires through the wheelchair provider or at a bike shop.

10. Accessories (optional)

    a. Ask what is available.

    b. Arm rest

     i Some people feel it interferes with pushing and the style or sleekness they want.

     ii. Push handles can be attached or are part of the back of the frame.

    c. Anti-tip wheels are attached to the bottom of the back of the chair to help prevent tipping and may be required on some transport vehicles.

11. Specialized equipment attached to a chair requires individual training and manufacturer's guidelines. Add what care is required to your *Personal Care Handbook* and the *Personal Caregiver Handbook*.

12. It can be exciting once you find out that the item you have waited for finally arrives, so it is easy to overlook what may be very important. Therefore, be sure to check and review the following:

    a.   All the areas that are important for you and the order to ensure that you received the product you wanted the way you want it.

    b.   Proper balance and comfort

    c.   Ensure that the wheelchair will not tip backward easily. If it does, it may require the following:

        i   Anti-tip wheels to prevent falling. Check with the mobility specialist to ensure you are safe and comfortable.

        ii.   The wheel axle plate placement to adjust the chair balance

        iii.   The height of the caster wheels may need adjusting.

II. <u>Cushions</u>: General Information

1. It is very important to request an experienced seating specialist to assist you with proper seating evaluation assessments. You will need a prescription from your physician.

2. Generally, cushions are made of various materials. They can include a combination of products, such as foam, gel packs, honeycomb, and air cells. If you have an allergy to latex or another foam product, it will be very important to notify the service provider.

3. The purpose of a properly fitted back and seating cushion provides the following:

    a.   Balance and comfort

    b.   Better positioning and seating posture

    c.   To help prevent decubitus sores

    d.   To provide comfort as using the seating sling of the wheelchair can become uncomfortable when sitting for any length of time, making a properly fitted cushion necessary

4. *It is important to check* for any hard surfaces that may be touching any part of the back or buttock areas as it could create a sore. Discuss with your seating specialist or physician.

5. Cushion and wheelchair reevaluation

    a.   Check with your insurance provider regarding the replacement frequency for your equipment.

    b.   Generally, the reassessment can be a minimum of every two to three years or after a surgery that can affect your needs.

A. Seating Cushion

1. The purpose is for comfort, balance, leg and feet placement, and to help prevent decubitus sores.

2. Consult a seating specialist to evaluate if a special seating cushion is required to accommodate the needs caused by pressure areas or medical concerns.

3. Things to be considered in the evaluation:

    a. Request a pressure evaluation to ensure that the cushion recommended provides the best support. It may be necessary to evaluate various types of cushions.

    b. Shoulder placement. Are they balanced while using the chair? Is the individual balanced in all aspects of the chair and its use?

    c. Be sure there is a two-finger space between the back of the knee and the edge of the cushion. This helps body-seating placement to prevent blood clots and leg pressure.

    d. Cushion height can increase the overall chair height. Consider table-height comfort when at a normal height table for meals, work, and school; in the car, you need to consider the roof if the head is touching, etc.

4. Be sure cushion cover is clean and fits correctly—no gaps or bulges.

    a. The manufacturer can supply additional zippered covers for an additional cost.

    b. You can purchase material and have a cover made with elastic so it is easy to change and wash. Not only is this economical, but it is also nice when the material is personalized.

    c. The removable seat cover should be changed at least once a day or when soiled. Note: It may appear clean, but you could notice a strong odor.

    d. White vinegar acts as an antibacterial to help remove odor and to clean with laundry.

5. In cleaning a soiled cushion, consider the following:

    a. *Check the manufacturer's booklet for their cleaning recommendations.*

    b. *Do not wash unless it is stated on the cushion.*

    c. Most cushions have a removable zippered cover. Clean as directed.

    d. If there are no instructions available and no removable cover, you can gently clean with soft cloth.

        i. Use mild soap, adding a little white vinegar to your water. White vinegar acts as an antibacterial to help remove odor and clean.

        ii. Baking soda also can help with cleaning and odor. Note: Do not use the baking soda and the vinegar together as it can undesirably produce foam that is similar to a science experiment. There are cleaning products specially designed to minimize or eliminate odor available through medical suppliers.

            • You can check with your insurance for coverage when you place an order for incontinent products.

- These products are generally designed for any *plastic*, such as tubing or any type of leg bags as it minimizes breaking down of the product.
    iii. Remove most of the moisture with a damp cloth.
    iv. Pat dry with towel and use a hair dryer if needed.
6. Cushion or wheelchair odor
   a. This can be embarrassing for the person using the chair. It would be best to find the source and clean as soon as possible.
   b. In the event you experience a problem when you are away from your home, you can maintain the dignity of the individual from embarrassment by being prepared. Keeping something in the vehicle like the following can help:
  - Additional covers and clothing
  - Lysol spray to disinfect
  - Unscented air freshener or cologne
  - Or something you may find that works better

B. **Back cushion**. Generally, this is special ordered through a seating specialist.
1. The purpose of this is for back protection, lower back support, balance, and seating comfort.
2. Be sure that it fits properly and attached appropriately.

III. <u>**Shower Chair**</u>
1. It is recommended to install a handheld showerhead for an individual with a disability. There are several selections available. Check to see which one is best for your needs. The one with a water control on the nozzle makes it easier and generally preferred by most individuals.
2. There are a variety of styles of shower chairs that can meet your needs. Be sure you find one that provides stability, safety, and balance.
3. Be careful of the chairs without a back support or lightweight chairs as they do not provide the stability and balance support most often needed that may make it more of a safety hazard.
4. For showering in a bathtub, it is recommended to have a sturdy, long, padded chair with a back support that allows for stability and better balance. This fits over the side of a bathtub, allowing easier access.
5. If staying at a hotel, call ahead and ask what type of shower chair they have available to ensure that it will meet your individual needs for balance, stability, and safety.

6. Take a portable travel shower chair to ensure stability when away from home. There are portable shower chairs available online that are lightweight and easy to transport. Taking your own chair helps to ensure stability, safety, comfort, and independence.

7. You may need to use both the hotel's shower chair and your portable shower chair depending on the accessibility needed for transferring or for an additional seating area.

IV. **Bags**. See Personal Bags Organization section for more information.

1. A backpack should generally carry personal supplies and spare clothes.

2. A side pack or an under-chair pack holds the following personal belongings:
   a. Wallet
   b. Keys
   c. Etc.

3. Phone pack
   a. Attach to the side of chair
   b. Phone bag should be waterproof type.
   c. Has a closure to minimize any water exposure
   d. Phone is always charged and ready for usage (the caregiver to check.)

V. **Accessories.** Look on the Internet for wheelchairs, cushions, and accessories.

1. Emergency alert button (optional)
   a. Check the equipment as stated on the instruction sheet.
   b. Check periodically to be sure it works and if it requires new batteries or charging.

VI. **Customized Vehicles and Vans with a Lift**

1. There are several service dealers available. You will need to check in your area.

2. Be careful with the door height to ensure that the person sitting in the chair can fit through the height opening; an expanded top may be required.

3. Vehicles can be equipped with hand controls. A therapist can assist with more information.

4. It will be important to work with a driver training instruction specialist for disabled individuals to understand how to drive with the adaptive equipment safely.

5. It would be best to understand how to repair some of the equipment and what to do if a problem occurs (i.e., the lift will not move, etc.)

6. When purchasing a new vehicle many times, a dealership may provide a credit for adaptive equipment. Check with your dealership on the dollar allowance and if they will do the modification.

VII. **Miscellaneous Equipment**

1. It would be best to speak with your physician, occupational and physical therapist, and the mobility provider regarding equipment to best assist you and what is recommended for your mobility and safety, such as the following:

    a. Walker; there are many styles. Check with your mobility provider or therapist as one style may appear more portable or offer additional benefits, but it may not be the right one. It may be a safety hazard that you are not aware of and can affect your balance.

    b. There are many types of products available, and it would be helpful to research the product for your specific needs. Your local medical supplier will have booklets and products for you to consider.

2. If you have very specialized equipment, you may want to have the booklet or copy a specific page from the manual that best explains the equipment and the care needed.

3. Keeping the various equipment manuals in a central location for easy access will make it easier to reference should the need arise if a breakdown occurs.

VIII. **Additional Equipment and Information**

List all your equipment that you want a caregiver to understand how it is maintained and its purpose. Add additional information needed for your individual needs and living style.

_____

_____

_____

_____

_____

_____

_____

_____

_____

_____

_____

_____

Equipment Maintenance

Fill in

CONTACT 1. Primary caregiver ❑ See list _____ Phone _____

          2. Mobility service provider _____ Contact _____

             Phone _____ E-mail _____

             Address _____

             _____

The individual and the primary caregiver should take time before an item is purchased to understand the purpose and the need for the equipment. *Make a copy of this form for each item.*

I. **Item**_____ Date _____

    1. Purpose

        a. _____

        b. _____

        c. _____

    2. Do you need a prescription? ❑ YES ❑ NO

        a. Doctor_____ Phone _____

        b. _____

    3. Funding ❑ Insurance ❑ Regional Center ❑ Self ❑ Other

        a. Purchase coverage _____

        b. Co-pay _____

        c. Frequency of replacement _____

    4. Who handles any repairs?

        a. _____

    5. What are the safety considerations? ❑ See attached

        a. _____

        b. _____

    6. Maintenance and care ❑ See attached

        a. _____

        b. _____

        c. _____

    7. Accessories (optional)

        a. _____

        b. _____

c. _____

8. Description ❑ See attached

Color_____ Fabric_____ Height_____ Length_____ Width_____ Weight_____

a. _____

b. _____

9. Transportation (if applicable)

❑ Fits in current vehicle ❑ Modifications to vehicle required ❑ New vehicle required

❑ Meets public transportation standards

a. _____

b. _____

10. ❑ Reevaluation assessments ❑ Repair ❑ Other _____

a. Date_____

Comment_____

_____

b. Date_____

Comment_____

_____

c. Date_____

Comment_____

_____

II. Cushion or Seating

A. Seating cushion

a. Date_____

❑ Replace ❑ Repair ❑ Cleaning frequency_____

_____

b. Date_____

❑ Replace ❑ Repair ❑ Cleaning frequency_____

_____

2. Special Instructions ❑ See attached

a. Check the manufacturer's booklet for their cleaning recommendations.

b. ❑ Wash removable cover_____

c. ❑ Cleaning instructions_____

d. ❑ _____

Note: Add additional information needed for your individual needs and living style.

12
Intake Log

It can be important to chart the amount of fluids and meals an individual is consuming. Depending on the medical condition, this information can be helpful for the primary caregiver. It can ensure the diet is appropriate and to be able to share with the medical team who may want to make some adjustments or recommendations to enhance the appropriate diet.

Intake Log

Monitor all food and liquid intake.

Date	Morning			Noon			Night			Total Daily Ounces
	Amount	Type	Ounces	Amount	Type	Ounces	Amount	Type	Ounces	
Mon										
TOTAL										
Tues										
TOTAL										
Wed										
TOTAL										
Thurs										
TOTAL										
Fri										
TOTAL										
Sat										
TOTAL										
Sun										
TOTAL										

Measure the bowl or the cup/glass you are using with a measuring cup to determine the exact measurement.

13
Laundry

The caregiver will be handling the laundry and you want to ensure they do it to your specifications. It will be important to have some instructions for them to follow. You can post your instructions on a cabinet or wall in your laundry room; or, have the information available if they have go to a laundry room in your complex or laundromat, and ensure they have the appropriate money/coins.

Every washer and dryer is a little different to use, so be sure you give instructions on how to use your machines. Don't assume everyone washes or dry's clothes the same as you and will know how to use your machines. Therefore, it is important to explain verbally and have written instructions:

1. The way you prefer to wash and dry.
2. How to separate the laundry,
3. What is dried in the dryer or hung to dry? If hung to dry, where do they hang the clothes.
4. Laundry products:
    a. Type of different laundry products you use for a specific wash load.
    b. The amount of each product.
    c. When to use a certain product; i.e.
        i.   Laundry detergent.
        ii.   Bleach on whites only.
        iii. White vinegar on towels and items soiled from incontinence.
        iv.   Fabric softener.
5. Water temperature depending on the type of load.
6. Dryer heat temperature depending on the type of load.
7. You may have additional instructions.

Also, it is important what items MUST go to the laundry service for dry cleaning. It is surprising how some people wash everything and do not read the labels to see if they require special handling.

A few examples of things going poorly and resulting in damaged clothing.
1. A wool sweater gets washed and dried in the dryer. The sweater has now shrunk to a smaller size.
2. Adding bleach to everything will help sanitize the wash. However, bleach will whiten dark clothing or cause white spots on the item.

3. A person is not accustomed to sending clothing for dry cleaning. They wash and dry everything including dress suits and the ties.

Remember to keep your dry-cleaning items separate from your washing items. Having instructions will not only help your caregiver but help save on having to purchase new items.

LAUNDRY INSTRUCTIONS
Sample

IMPORTANT:

Be sure to check the label of each item in the event there is special washing, drying, or require dry cleaning and need to go to a laundry service.

SEPARATE CLOTHES:

1. Towels, protective covers
2. Clothes, sheets
    a. White shirts may need to be separated depending on the type of dark clothes, especially if introducing a new dark or red clothing item.
    b. Protective covers can be added

LOAD SIZE: **LARGE -** Depending on how much loaded

TEMPERATURE: ❑ Warm Water ❑ Cold Water

FILL WASH TUB

1. <u>Towels, protective covers</u>
    a. 1 cup of laundry soap put in tub
    b. 2 cups of white vinegar – works as a disinfectant & neutralizes the Ph from the urine.
    c. ¼ cup of fabric softener. Not too much, but allows for a nice smell to the towels.

2. <u>Clothes, sheets</u>
    a. 1 cup of laundry soap put in tub
    b. 2 cups of white vinegar – works as a disinfectant & neutralizes the Ph from the urine.
    c. ½ to 1 cup of fabric softener depending on load size

DRYER

1. Full dry cycle
2. Heat – high

*IMPORTANT – CLEAN OUT LINT FILTER AFTER EVERY LOAD

Do not wash:

1. Any item you have a question or doubtful. Ask before washing.
2. Cushions
3. Suits or ties
4. Any items that states on the label to dry clean.

14
Meal Suggestions

It is very helpful to have meal suggestions for the caregiver. The individual can always make a request for something different. However, the caregiver can easily make suggestions from the list provided. Many times, the caregiver can be of a different nationality, and they may not be familiar to the prepared meals the way you are accustomed to making.

Try to have your suggestions easy to follow. If there is a special meal that may be a little complex to prepare, you may want to prepare it in advance, and they can serve it.

Check with your caregiver on their culinary skills with preparing a meal. It is best not to assume a person knows how to make even the simplest sandwich or even fry an egg.

Meal Suggestions

Provides helpful meal suggestions.

If the individual has sensitive food allergies, take a copy when admitted into the hospital to assist the dietician with suggestions.

FOOD ALLERGIES		
Allergy	**Reaction**	**Note: Include a remedy**

Meals   **Suggestions:** *Ask the primary caregiver or the individual for daily preference.* **Please minimize frying and high-fat content of foods. Bake or use microwave preferably.**
<u>Breakfast</u>
<u>Lunch</u>
<u>Dinner</u>
<u>Drinks</u>   water
<u>NOTE</u>

15
Medical Concerns Checklist

When an illness or medical condition occurs, this section describes how the caregiver can best assist the individual. It is also helpful for the medical team when an emergency arises. It will be important that all information is thoroughly documented and kept up to date.

As the origin of the needs attached to the sample form pertain mostly to an individual with spina bifida, it may have areas that do not pertain to your specific needs. Simply change any or all areas to meet your individual needs.

Take this with you when an emergency occurs or if there is a medical situation that you have been having a problem to find a solution. This form has been well received and helpful to the medical team, especially in an emergency when they are working to eliminate a diagnosis to find the appropriate treatment. It has eliminated specific testing and expedited in locating a treatment.

It also gives the medical team the confidence of the "team approach," and they generally welcome your ideas and assistance easier.

I have provided a sample of various conditions with symptom, what to look for, and of common situations that can occur. You will need to note the situation of the various conditions individually as each individual is unique, and their symptoms and what to do are different.

Medical Concerns Checklist

Sample Form

Name_____ Date_____

CONTACT 1. Primary caregiver ❑ See list_____ Phone_____

           2. Physician ❑ See list_____ Phone_____

> ➢ *Notify* the primary caregiver or the physician immediately if you notice an illness, condition, or abnormality.

WHEN AN ILLNESS OR CONDITION OCCURS, HERE ARE AREAS TO CONSIDER.

There are separate sections regarding each area with more explicit information to assist you.

A. Remember: If you need to go to the doctor or the emergency room, take the following:

    a. *Personal Medical Journal* or medical history summary

    b. Medical supply bag with the individual's specific incontinence and/or personal items, especially nonlatex items if there is a latex allergy

    c. List of all current prescription, herbal supplements, over-the-counter medication

    d. List of all allergies to medication and special medications used for various radiology testing

    e. *Personal Caregiver Handbook* that includes specific personal information or the Medical Concerns Checklist

    f. Any X-rays to assist a medical professional that is located_____

IMPORTANT: DO NOT LEAVE ANY X-RAYS OR REPORTS AT THE HOSPITAL OR AT PHYSICIAN'S OFFICE!

B. Vomiting. Always be alert for other symptoms that may be part of this situation.

    a. _____

    b. _____

C. Blood Pressure and Heart Rate

    a. Normal is approximately 120/80. Individual's normal is_____.

    b. If elevated, check all areas in this Medical Concerns Checklist section for possible reasons for the elevation.

D. Fever. Notify the primary caregiver and/or the physician immediately.

    a. Individual's normal temperature is approximately_____.

    b. Anything above normal warrants checking for a medical condition, such as a urinary tract infection (UTI), decubitus, broken bones, infections, etc.

    c. _____

E. Travel. When going to the doctor or hospital, see the Community Transportation section.

a. If you have latex allergies, take all nonlatex products in your medical travel bag with personal items, any applicable *X-rays*, and notebook or binder with caregiver notes, especially the Daily Vitals Record Keeping that includes the blood pressure and temperature.

F. Concern Areas. The following areas have corresponding numbers to the pages that provide additional pertinent information:

1. **Allergies** ❑ Medication ❑ Food ❑ _____ See Page___
2. **Decubitus** See Page___
3. **Seizures** See Page___
4. **Shunts** See Page___
5. **Stroke Identification** See Page___
6. **Urinary Tract Infection** See Page___
7. **Vomiting** See Page___
8. _____ See Page___
9. _____ See Page___
10. _____ See Page___
11. _____ See Page___
12. _____ See Page___
13. _____ See Page___
14. _____ See Page___

1. <u>Allergies</u>

<u>CONTACT</u> 1. Primary caregiver ❑ See list _____ Phone _____

2. Physician ❑ See list _____ Phone _____

➢ *Notify* the primary caregiver or the physician immediately if you notice an illness, condition, or abnormality.

• **See Medication and Food Allergy List.** If additional information is needed, add another sheet.

i. <u>**Medication**</u> ❑ See additional list.

A. TYPE_____

1. Symptom_____

2. Remedy

a. Medication_____

b. How to assist_____

c. _____

B. TYPE

1. Symptom_____

2. Remedy

a. Medication_____

b. How to assist_____

c. _____

ii. <u>**Foods**</u> ❑ See additional list.

A. TYPE_____

1. Symptom_____

2. Remedy

a. Medication_____

b. How to assist_____

c. _____

B. TYPE_____

1. Symptom_____

2. Remedy

a. Medication_____

b. How to assist_____

c. _____

2. Decubitus - Bed Sores - Burns

CONTACT 1. Primary caregiver ❑ See list _____ Phone _____

2. Physician ❑ See list _____ Phone _____

➢ *Notify* the primary caregiver or the physician immediately if you notice an illness, condition, or abnormality.

• The physician will need to see the patient and may refer care to a wound care specialist.

A. Symptoms

a. Vomiting

b. Fever

c. Open wound

d. Skin discoloration at wound site

e. Other (Explain)_____

B. Check Body

a. Feet, especially for burn blisters (i.e., water too hot in shower, infections, or poor circulation)

b. Legs, especially for burn blisters (i.e., water too hot in shower, placing hot items on thighs, prolonged computer laptop use if resting on legs, exposure to sun, any type of open wound, or infection)

c. Buttock area for discoloration, any type of open wound, or infection

d. Arm and elbow area for possible sores or burn blisters

e. Fingers for possible blisters, any injuries, or sores from pushing a wheelchair, walker, etc.

f. Private area for an infection, yeast infection, or decubitus ulcers

g. Bruises, open wounds

h. Other (Explain)_____

C. Wounds

a. Be sure to follow the instructions of your physician or the wound care specialist.

b. When you first identify a wound, be sure to cover with some type of light bandage.

c. Do not put any pressure on the wound area.

d. Monitor the wound area when sitting or lying and observe how the body comes in contact with any pressure area.

e. Check with your insurance carrier; you may have medical coverage for wound care supplies. You will have to obtain a prescription from your physician in most cases. Be sure to ask where to obtain supplies.

f. Assess what wound supplies you may have at home in case a new or reorder is necessary.

g. When calling the medical supplier, be sure to mention you are handling a wound and need the order quickly.

D. **Cleaning of Wound Area**

a. Follow the direction of your physician or wound care specialist.

E. **General Information**

a. Remember there should be no hard contact with the injured area.

b. Use a light sheet to cover if the wound is on the buttock or private area to maintain the dignity of the individual.

c. Ask the specialist for all other instructions, such as if they can take a shower, travel, sit, etc.

F. **Progression of wound healing generally observed**. Check with the specialist for more information.

a. White layer

b. Pink layer

c. Bloody (good - means circulation is established)

d. Edges become smaller

e. Repeat of numbers 1–4 above until healed

f. Continually prompt and monitor to stay off the area.

g. Ask your physician if the following would be recommended:

- An increase level of zinc has been known to improve skin redevelopment (be sure to discuss with physician prior to increasing zinc so there is no conflict with treatment, medication, or blood levels. Zinc can be taken orally or used topically).

- Protein food or nutrients have been recognized as a good source for tissue redevelopment.

G. **Latex Allergy and Other Allergies**

a. If you have latex allergies, take all nonlatex products in your medical bag with personal items.

b. Be sure to take your nonallergy products that include tape, gloves, etc.

H. **Follow-up**

a. Everyone who is working with the client will need to have the instructions for the proper care from the doctor or wound care specialist and from your notes.

b. Visiting nursing staff may be required to come in periodically to check the wound and dressing and make any recommendations.

I. **Prevention Techniques**

    a. Cushions for wheelchairs and other seating devices:

        1. Fitting is appropriate.

        2. Placement is appropriate.

            a. Back

- Should be secured to back of chair and not worn down
- See Equipment Maintenance section for proper seating, fitting, and maintenance.

            b. Seat

- Should not show excessive wear
- Should not have a hard or uneven surface that could create a decubitus sore

        3. Fabric

            a. Securely on cushions

            b. Changed and washed daily or when soiled

        4. Transfers. Watch how individual transfers in and out of chair.

            a. Is the body hitting or rubbing anything that could create a sore?

            b. Be sure to advise the client as they may not realize they are creating a sore or understand the importance of an alternative transfer method.

        5. Bedding. Monitor the bedding to ensure it is free of wrinkles and bulk, secured well, and the bottom area of the bedding is flat.

        6. Clothing. Watch for bulk created by seams, zippers, pockets, waist bands, and type of pant fabric, etc.

3. Seizures

CONTACT 1. Primary caregiver ❑ See list _____ Phone _____

2. Physician ❑ See list _____ Phone _____

> ➢ *Notify* the primary caregiver or the physician immediately if you notice an illness, condition, or abnormality.

★ Note: *Do not give* any Tylenol, aspirin, or ibuprofen type medication. This can mask a symptom if there is a serious medical condition.

A. **Symptoms.** These are some symptoms to be able to distinguish a seizure. You may have other information as symptoms are different for each individual:

  a. Discoloration of skin, purplish or whitish

  b. Disoriented

    1. Speech sluggish, or verbiage is not clear

    2. Unable to stay with a conversation

    3. Appears on some type of drug

  c. Eyes fixed or strange movements

  d. Shaking of the body

  e. If the person has a shunt, it could represent an additional problem.

B. **Concerns**

  a. Check each area of the Medical Concerns Checklist section for possibilities of medical problems that could cause the seizure.

  b. It could be the possibility of medication reaction that affects blood levels.

  c. When taking to doctor or hospital, see the Community Transportation section.

  d. If you have latex allergies, take all nonlatex products, medical travel bag with personal items, any applicable *X-rays*, and notebook or binder with caregiver notes, especially the Daily Vital Record Keeping that includes the blood pressure and temperature.

C. **Follow-up**

Everyone working with the individual will need to have the instructions on how to handle future seizures.

D. **Additional Information**

_____

_____

_____

_____

_____

_____

4. **Shunts** – The following information pertains to hydrocephalus (be sure to add another type of shunts and explain the location and any pertinent information to ensure another person will know what symptoms to consider if a situation occurs).

<u>**CONTACT**</u> 1. Primary caregiver ❑ See list _____ Phone _____
                 2. Physician ❑ See list _____ Phone _____
        ➢ *Notify* the primary caregiver or the physician immediately if you notice an illness, condition, or abnormality.

A. **Symptoms.** It will be best to list the symptoms you want to ensure are monitored by your physician.

     ❑ Headache   ❑ Eye sensitivity to light   ❑ Cognitive speech is unclear

     ❑ Red mark or line tracking on neck and chest areas   ❑ Swelling around tubing area

     ❑ The ophthalmologist can check to see if there is pressure on the optic nerve.

     ❑ _____

     ❑ _____

     ❑ _____

     ❑ _____

B. **How to handle:** *Do not pump the shunt* unless instructed by the neurosurgeon. Overpumping can drain the brain of fluid. Explain what information is important for your caregiver to understand when symptoms occur.

_____

_____

_____

_____

_____

_____

_____

_____

_____

_____

_____

5. <u>Stroke Identification</u>

If he or she has trouble with *any one* of the following tasks, call emergency immediately and describe.

Sometimes symptoms of a stroke are difficult to identify. Unfortunately, the lack of awareness spells disaster. The stroke victim may suffer severe brain damage when people fail to recognize the symptoms of a stroke.

Now doctors say you can recognize a stroke by asking *three* simple questions:

<u>**S**</u> - Ask the individual to *smile.*

<u>**T**</u> - Ask the person to *talk* and *speak a simple sentence* (coherently), for example, "It is sunny out today," and the person is unable to stay focused in a conversation.

<u>**R**</u> - Ask them to *raise both arms.*

Another sign of a stroke – "Stick out your tongue"
- Ask the person to "stick" out his/her tongue.
- If the tongue is crooked or if it goes to one side or the other, that is also an indication of a stroke.

You may want to include additional information.

This is a situation that could have been prevented.

During a BBQ, a woman stumbled and took a little fall. She assured everyone that she was fine (they offered to call paramedics). She said she had just tripped over a brick because of her new shoes.

They got her cleaned up and got her a new plate of food. While she appeared a bit shaken up, Jane went about enjoying herself the rest of the evening.

Jane's husband called later, telling everyone that his wife had been taken to the hospital. At 6:00 p.m., Jane passed away. She had suffered a stroke at the BBQ.

Had they known how to identify the signs of a stroke, perhaps Jane would be with us today. Some don't die. They can end up in a helpless, hopeless condition instead.

A neurologist says that if he can get to a stroke victim within three hours, he can hopefully reverse the effects of a stroke *totally*. He said the trick was getting a stroke recognized and diagnosed and then getting the patient medically cared for within three hours, which can be the difficult part.

This information is to assist you and a collection from several sources.

6. **Urinary Tract Infection (UTI)**

CONTACT   1.   Primary caregiver ❑ See list _____ Phone _____

           2.   Physician ❑ See list _____ Phone _____

➢ *Notify* the primary caregiver or the physician immediately if you notice an illness, condition, or abnormality.

A. **Symptoms**

    a. Blood in urine (pain, spasms, or discomfort)

    b. Smell, strong odor (can indicate an infection)

        1. Noticeable as soon as you enter the room or surroundings

        2. Stools will also have a stronger odor

    c. Vomiting

    d. Fever

    e. Irritability

    f. Blood pressure increase or decrease

    g. Lethargy

    h. Back pain on either the left or right side may generally indicate a kidney infection.

B. **Urine Analysis (UA)**

    a. Bloody

    b. It is important to take a urine sample to the doctor's office or a designated laboratory to establish the type of bacteria for the proper diagnosis and medication to ensure the appropriate treatment.

    c. Write instructions of how to obtain urine sample, which would be best handled for the individual, or the physician will be able to give you explicit instructions to follow.

      • The (UA) urine specimen container should be placed in a baggie to prevent leakage with individual's name and date.

      • The UA can be placed in a brown lunch bag with the name on the outside.

      • Then it should be placed in the refrigerator or placed on ice to prevent bacteria growth until taken immediately from the refrigerator to the physician or laboratory. Ask the maximum length of time to be kept refrigerated before dropping it off and any other considerations to handle the specimen.

C. **Make an appointment as soon as possible.**

    a. Be sure to pack any incontinence products to include latex-free products if applicable:

      • Diapers (briefs), pads, and/or catheters

      • Gloves

- Wallet with insurance card, credit card, checkbook, or cash to pay the doctor
- Assist as needed

Note: A transportation service can require twenty-four-hour notice.

D. **Follow-up**. Find out if there is a bacterial infection and what treatment is recommended.

a. The doctor will give instructions as to what is needed. Be sure to ask when the results will be available.

b. It will be important to follow up with a phone call or to check online for the results. Do not depend on a call back from the doctor's office.

c. If a prescription is necessary,

1. check against the allergy listing,
2. give the doctor's office your pharmacy number or location _____,
3. pick up the medication.

d. When you pick up the medication, check to ensure it is what has been prescribed by the physician.

1. It is recommended to keep all medication in a medication tray to ensure it is distributed appropriately.
2. Notify the *primary caregiver immediately* upon onset of any complications or if you notice the medication appears to be correcting the symptoms in a timely manner.

E. **Recheck**. Be sure to ask the doctor if they need any of the following:

a. To have another urinalysis to ensure the infection has been eliminated

b. Another appointment. If so,

1. schedule the appointment and
2. contact your transportation service if applicable.

F. **Additional Information**

_____
_____
_____
_____
_____
_____
_____
_____
_____
_____
_____

7. <u>Vomiting</u>

❑ This can be an indication of other concerns that need to be checked, such as the flu or another diagnosis.

<u>CONTACT</u>   1. Primary caregiver ❑ See list _____ Phone _____
2. Physician ❑ See list _____ Phone _____

➤ *Notify* the primary caregiver or the physician immediately if you notice an illness, condition, or abnormality.

A. **Symptoms.** Always be alert for other symptoms that may be a trigger of this situation.

a. Depending on the disability, vomiting could be a trigger indicating the individual is having a medical concern that could be more serious. It will be important to monitor and check to ensure you have eliminated all medical issues that may be involved.

Note: If a person is unable to speak or is paralyzed, they may not be able to tell you when there is a medical issue that needs attention. Their body could react by vomiting, giving you the alert to examine all areas of the individual to locate the source of the problem.

Medical concerns that are triggered with vomiting as the first indication there is a problem:

_____   _____
_____   _____
_____   _____

It will be important to monitor the following to make the decision if you need to contact the physician or take to the nearest hospital emergency. Frequency of vomiting creates dehydration, which can be very serious and require intravenous (IV) fluids.

1. Frequency _____
2. Color ❑ Food ❑ Blood ❑ Phlegm
3. ❑ Note _____

_____
_____

B. **How to handle**

❑ Call doctor_____

❑ Emergency   ❑ Immediately   ❑ Monitor_____

❑ Medication   Type_____ Dosage_____ Frequency_____

❑ Other_____

_____

_____

_____

8. Other_____

CONTACT 1. Primary caregiver ❑ See list _____ Phone _____

            2. Physician ❑ See list _____ Phone _____

      ➤ *Notify* the primary caregiver or the physician immediately if you notice an illness, condition, or abnormality.

❑ See additional sections with more information.

A. **Symptoms**

    ❑ _____

    ❑ _____

    ❑ _____

    ❑ _____

    ❑ _____

    ❑ _____

B. **How to handle. ❑ Seek medical attention immediately.**

_____

_____

_____

_____

_____

_____

_____

_____

_____

_____

_____

_____

_____

_____

_____

_____

Fill-In Form: It will be important that all information is thoroughly documented and kept up to date. This form is for you to customize to meet your needs.

Medical Concerns Checklist

Name_____Date_____

CONTACT 1. Primary caregiver ❑ See list _____ Phone _____
            2. Physician ❑ See list _____ Phone _____
   ➢ *Notify* the primary caregiver or the physician immediately if you notice an illness, condition, or abnormality.

WHEN AN ILLNESS OR CONDITION OCCURS, HERE ARE AREAS TO CONSIDER.

There are separate sections regarding each area with more explicit information to assist you.

A. **Remember:** If you need to go to the doctor or the emergency room, take the following:

   a. *Personal Medical Journal* or medical history summary

   b. Medical supply bag with the individual's specific incontinence and/or personal items, especially nonlatex items if there is a latex allergy

   c. *Personal Caregiver Handbook* that includes specific personal information or the Medical Concerns Checklist

   d. Any X-rays to assist a medical professional that is located _____

IMPORTANT: DO NOT LEAVE ANY X-RAYS OR REPORTS AT THE HOSPITAL OR AT PHYSICIAN'S OFFICE!

B. **Vomiting.** Always be alert for other symptoms that may be part of this situation.

   a. _____

   b. _____

C. **Blood Pressure and Heart Rate**

   a. Normal is approximately 120/80. Individual's normal is _____.

   b. If elevated, check all areas in this Medical Concerns Checklist section for possible reasons for the elevation.

D. **Fever**. Notify the primary caregiver and/or the physician immediately.

   a. Individual's normal temperature is approximately _____.

   b. Anything above normal warrants checking for a medical condition, such as a urinary tract infection (UTI), decubitus, broken bones, infections, etc.

   c. _____

E. **Concern Areas.** The following areas have corresponding numbers to the pages that provides additional pertinent information:

1. **Allergies** ❑ Medication ❑ Food ❑ _____ See Page___
2. **Decubitus** _____ See Page___
3. **Seizures** _____ See Page___
4. **Shunts** _____ See Page___
5. **Stroke Identification** _____ See Page___
6. **Urinary Tract Infection** _____ See Page___
7. **Vomiting** _____ See Page___
8. _____ See Page___

1. **<u>Allergies</u>**

<u>**CONTACT**</u> 1. Primary caregiver ❑ See list _____ Phone _____

           2. Physician ❑ See list _____ Phone _____

      ➢ *Notify* the primary caregiver or the physician immediately if you notice an illness, condition, or abnormality.

        ➢ **SEE MEDICATION AND FOOD ALLERGY LIST.** If additional information is needed, add another sheet.

A. **<u>Medication</u>** ❑ See additional list.

    a. TYPE

       1. Symptom_____

       2. Remedy

          a. Medication _____

          b. How to assist _____

          c. _____

    b. TYPE

       1. Symptom _____

       2. Remedy

          a. Medication _____

          b. How to assist _____

          c. _____

B. **<u>Foods</u>** ❑ See additional list.

    a. TYPE

       1. Symptom_____

       2. Remedy

          a. Medication _____

          b. How to assist _____

          c. _____

    b. TYPE

       1. Symptom_____

       2. Remedy

          a. Medication _____

          b. How to assist _____

          c. _____

2. **Decubitus, Bedsores, Burns**

CONTACT   1. Primary caregiver ❑ See list _____ Phone _____

           2. Physician ❑ See list _____ Phone _____

➢ *Notify* the primary caregiver or the physician immediately if you notice an illness, condition, or an abnormality.

➢ The physician will need to see the patient and may refer care to a wound care specialist.

A. **Symptoms**

    a. _____

    b. _____

    c. _____

    d. _____

B. **Examine the body**

    a. _____

    b. _____

    c. _____

    d. _____

C. **Wounds**

    a. _____

    b. _____

    c. _____

    d. _____

D. **Cleaning of wound area**

    a. _____

    b. _____

    c. _____

    d. _____

E. **General information**

    a. _____

    b. _____

    c. _____

    d. _____

F. **Notes**

_____

_____

_____

_____

_____

_____

_____

G. **Progression of wound healing generally observed.** Check with the specialist for more information.

1. White layer

2. Pink layer

3. Bloody (good - means circulation is established)

4. Edges become smaller

5. Repeat of numbers 1–4 above until healed

6. Continually prompt and monitor to stay off the area.

7. Ask your physician if the following would be recommended:

   • Increased levels of zinc have been known to improve skin redevelopment (be sure to discuss with physician prior to increasing zinc so there is no conflict with treatment or medication. Zinc can be taken orally or used topically.).

   • Protein food or nutrients have been recognized as a good source for tissue redevelopment.

H. **Medical appointment or travel.** When going to the doctor or hospital, see Community Transportation, section 6.

a. If you have latex allergies, take your nonlatex wound care products in your medical travel bag, including any personal items in the event a change of clothing or there is an incontinence issue, caregiver notes, and especially the current Daily Vitals Record Keeping Log.

I. **Follow-up**

a. _____

_____

b. _____

_____

J. **Prevention techniques**

a. Cushions for wheelchairs and other seating devices:

   1. Fitting is appropriate.

   2. Placement is appropriate.

      a. Back

         • _____

         • _____

b. Seat

- _____

- _____

3. Fabric

- _____

- _____

4. Transfers: Watch how individual transfers in and out of chair.

- _____

- _____

5. Bedding: Monitor the bedding to ensure it is free of wrinkles and bulk, secured well, and the bottom area of the bedding is flat.

- _____

- _____

6. Clothing: Watch for bulk created by seams, zippers, pockets, waist bands, and type of pant fabric, etc.

- _____

- _____

3. <u>Seizures</u>

<u>**CONTACT**</u> 1. Primary caregiver ❏ See list _____ Phone _____

2. Physician ❏ See list _____ Phone _____

➢ *Notify* the primary caregiver or the physician immediately if you notice an illness, condition, or an abnormality.

★ Note: *Do not give* any Tylenol, aspirin, or ibuprofen type of pain medication. This can mask a symptom if there is a serious medical condition.

A. **Symptoms**

- _____
- _____
- _____
- _____

B. **Concerns**

- _____
- _____
- _____

C. **Description of the seizures**

- _____
- _____
- _____
- _____
- _____
- _____

D. **During seizure concerns**

- _____
- _____
- _____

E. **Follow-up**

- _____
- _____
- _____

F. **Additional information**

- _____
- _____
- _____

4. **Shunts**

❑ See additional sections with more information.

CONTACT 1. Primary caregiver ❑ See list _____ Phone _____

                  2. Physician ❑ See list _____ Phone _____

      ➢ *Notify* the primary caregiver or the physician immediately if you notice an illness, condition, or abnormality.

A. **Symptoms.** It will be best to list the symptoms you want to ensure that they are monitored by your physician.

    ❑ Headache ❑ Eye sensitivity to light ❑ Sensitivity to noise ❑ Cognitive speech is unclear

    ❑ Red tracking on neck and chest areas ❑ Swelling around tubing area

    ❑ The ophthalmologist can check to see if there is pressure on the optic nerve.

    ❑ _____

    ❑ _____

    ❑ _____

    ❑ _____

B. **How to handle.** *Do not pump* **the shunt unless instructed by the neurosurgeon. Overpumping can drain the brain of fluid.**

_____

_____

_____

_____

_____

_____

_____

_____

_____

_____

_____

_____

5. <u>Stroke Identification</u>

If he or she has trouble with *any one* of the following tasks, call emergency immediately and describe the symptoms to the dispatcher.

Sometimes symptoms of a stroke are difficult to identify. Unfortunately, the lack of awareness spells disaster. The stroke victim may suffer severe brain damage when people fail to recognize the symptoms of a stroke.

Now doctors say you can recognize a stroke by asking *three* simple questions:

S - Ask the individual to *smile.*

T - Ask the person to *talk* and *speak a simple sentence* (coherently), for example, "It is sunny out today," and the person is unable to stay focused in the conversation.

R - Ask them to *raise both arms.*

Another sign of a stroke: "Stick out your tongue"
- Ask the person to stick out his tongue.
- If the tongue is crooked or if it goes to one side or the other, that is also an indication of a stroke.

You may want to include additional information.

6. **Urinary Tract Infection (UTI)**

CONTACT   1. Primary caregiver ❑ See list _____ Phone _____

             2. Physician ❑ See list _____ Phone _____

      ➤ *Notify* the primary caregiver or the physician immediately if you notice an illness, condition, or abnormality.

A. **Symptoms**

    a. _____

    b. _____

    c. _____

    d. _____

    e. _____

    f. _____

B. **Urine Analysis (UA)**

    a. Doctor's office_____

    b. Laboratory_____

    c. How to obtain sample_____

        • _____

        • _____

        • _____

        • _____

        • _____

C. **Make an appointment as soon as possible.**

    a. Be sure to pack any incontinence products to include latex-free products if applicable.

        • _____

        • _____

        • _____

        • _____

        • _____

D. **Follow-up**. Find out if there is a bacterial infection and what treatment is recommended.

    a. If a prescription is necessary,

        1. check against the allergy listing

        2. give the doctor's office your pharmacy number or location_____ and

3. pick up the medication

b. When you pick up the medication, check to ensure it is what has been prescribed by the physician.

• _____

E. **Recheck**. Be sure to ask the doctor if they need the following:

1. Schedule follow-up appointment.

2. Contact the transportation service if applicable.

F. **Additional Information**

_____
_____
_____
_____
_____
_____
_____
_____
_____
_____
_____
_____
_____
_____
_____

7. **Vomiting**

❑ This can be an indication of other concerns that need to be checked, such as the flu or another diagnosis.

CONTACT 1. Primary caregiver ❑ See list _____ Phone _____

               2. Physician ❑ See list _____ Phone _____

> ➢ *Notify* the primary caregiver or the physician immediately if you notice an illness, condition, or abnormality.

A. **Symptoms.** Always be alert for other symptoms that may be a trigger of this situation.

    a. Depending on the disability, vomiting could be a trigger, indicating the individual is having a medical concern that could be more serious. It will be important to monitor and check to ensure you have eliminated all medical issues that may be involved.

Note: If a person is unable to speak or is paralyzed, they may not be able to tell you when there is a medical issue that needs attention. Their body could react by vomiting, giving you the alert to examine all areas of the individual to locate the source of the problem.

Medical concerns that are triggered with vomiting as the first indication there is a problem:

_____   _____

_____   _____

_____   _____

It will be important to monitor the following to make the decision if you need to contact the physician or take to the nearest hospital emergency. Frequency of vomiting creates dehydration, which can be very serious and require intravenous (IV) fluids.

1. Frequency _____

2. Color ❑ Food ❑ Blood ❑ Phlegm

3. ❑ Note _____

_____

_____

B. **How to handle**

❑ Call Doctor _____

❑ Emergency   ❑ Immediately   ❑ Monitor _____

❑ Medication   Type_____Dosage _____ Frequency _____

❑ Other _____

_____

_____

8. _____

❑ See additional sections with more information.

CONTACT   1.   Primary caregiver ❑ See list _____ Phone _____

         2.   Physician ❑ See list _____ Phone _____

      ➤ *Notify* the primary caregiver or the physician immediately if you notice an illness, condition, or abnormality.

A.   Symptoms

❑ _____

❑ _____

❑ _____

❑ _____

❑ _____

❑ _____

B.   How to handle

_____

_____

_____

_____

_____

_____

_____

_____

_____

_____

_____

_____

_____

_____

_____

_____

16
Medical Occurrence Log

- This form is used when a medical condition occurs to keep everyone abreast of a situation.
- To prevent future confusion, use one form per type of medical situation.
- This will maintain an independent frequency log of reoccurring events, such as urinary tract infections (UTIs), falls, seizures, etc.
- Take this with you to the doctor's office to show the frequency of a situation. This can assist your medical team to help find a diagnosis, the need for further testing, or medication to help prevent the occurrence of a specific problem.
- Keep additional blank copies available in the back of the binder.

Medical Occurrence Log

❑ Urinary Tract Infections (UTI) ❑ _____ ❑ _____
❑ _____ ❑ _____ ❑ _____

➢ This can be used when there is a specific health occurrence and keep the incident on a separate log by subject or title to assist a physician of the frequency (i.e., seizures, falling, UTIs, etc.)

➢ Always *document and alert* the primary caregiver or physician of a medical occurrence immediately.

DATE			
TIME			
TYPE (Allergy, seizure, etc.)			
EXPLAIN what occurred			
RX given			
Other			
Other			
Other			
REPORTED to			
REPORTED by			

17
Medication Daily Schedule and Chart

This is *very important* to keep up to date, especially when medication needs to be distributed by the caregiver. It is recommended to have more than one pillbox for each time frame depending on the medication distribution. Having a medication pillbox will help ensure that the correct medication is taken and can prevent missing a medication, taking the wrong medication, or taking more than prescribed. It can be easy to forget you have taken a medication and then take another dosage.

You may want to keep the medication bottles in a separate container that holds all the medication, along with the Medication Daily Schedule. This helps keep them in a safe place, out of reach from visitors, and in some cases, the person to whom they are prescribed as they may have a tendency to get into them; a person with cognitive issues or dementia can get confused and take their medication more than what is prescribed.

Keep a Medication Chart of all over-the-counter medication and herbal supplements. It will be easier to stay aware of what and when medications have been taken and discontinued, or there was an allergic reaction.

Some pharmacies offer a "Bubble Pak" type of system whereby they have all the medication separated by time. There could be an additional charge, but this is an alternative that you could ask your pharmacist.

As a caregiver of an individual requiring assistance, having a weekly medication tray is helpful to see if the medication has been taken and that the medication is set up correctly to avoid a mistake.

Be careful if you allow the individual who needs assistance to be in charge of the weekly medication pillbox. It is recommended to check the pillbox to ensure that the medication is taken correctly. Also, if you have them fill the pillbox, watch and check that the medication is distributed correctly.

If a medication has been discontinued because of an allergic reaction, be sure to note it and add it to your "allergy list." State what the reaction was and what medication or hospital emergency was needed to remedy the situation.

It is *very important* to keep the medication information up to date, especially when distributed by the caregiver.

Medication Chart

Keep a summary list of all medication, even over-the-counter and herbal supplements, when discontinued and specify if there was an allergic reaction.

Date	Medication	Purpose	Dosage and Frequency	Reaction	Stopped	Comments

Medication Daily Schedule

Place the time and date in appropriate box.

Medication _____ Date started _____

Time

				Other

Discontinued Date_____ ❑ Monthly prescription refill Rx #_____
Reason: ❑ Completed   ❑ Reaction: Be sure to add to Allergy Section - Medication.

Place the time and date in appropriate box.

Medication _____ Date started _____

Time

				Other

Discontinued Date_____ ❑ Monthly prescription refill Rx #_____
Reason: ❑ Completed   ❑ Reaction: Be sure to add to Allergy Section - Medication.

Place the time and date in appropriate box.

Medication _____ Date started _____

Time

				Other

Discontinued Date_____ ❑ Monthly prescription refill Rx #_____
Reason: ❑ Completed   ❑ Reaction: Be sure to add to Allergy Section - Medication.

Place the time and date in appropriate box.

Medication _____ Date started _____

Time

				Other

Discontinued Date_____ ❑ Monthly prescription refill Rx #_____
Reason: ❑ Completed   ❑ Reaction: Be sure to add to Allergy Section - Medication.

Place the time and date in appropriate box.

Medication _____ Date started _____

Time

				Other

Discontinued Date_____ ❑ Monthly prescription refill Rx #_____
Reason: ❑ Completed   ❑ Reaction: Be sure to add to Allergy Section - Medication.

Place the time and date in appropriate box.

Medication _____ Date started _____

Time

				Other

Discontinued Date_____ ❑ Monthly prescription refill Rx #_____
Reason: ❑ Completed   ❑ Reaction: Be sure to add to Allergy Section - Medication.

18
Monitoring Log

<u>Blood Pressure</u>   <u>Glucose</u>   <u>Other</u>

It is important for many individuals to have a log of essential data to monitor and to show the medical team. This can be an optional form as you can keep similar information in the Daily Vitals Record Keeping Log to be used as needed.

It is recommended to keep a separate log sheet for each medical situation you are monitoring.

Monitoring Log

This is an optional form as you can keep similar information in the Daily Vitals Record Keeping Log to be used as needed.

❏ BLOOD PRESSURE ❏ GLUCOSE ❏ OTHER
Keep Each Category on a Separate Page

Date	A.M.	P.M.	Date	A.M.	P.M.

19
Personal Bag Organization

This section helps to ensure all personal bags for the individual who requires assistance has the information or items needed daily, in an emergency, or when traveling. It helps avoid an embarrassment to have the correct supplies when needed.

It will be important as the caregiver to check the bags periodically to ensure they have the appropriate items needed, such as a backpack with the daily personal supplies that may be needed if the individual must go to the bathroom or a doctor appointment. If a person is incontinent, they require items to ensure they maintain their dignity and avoid embarrassment to being able to clean up when away from their home.

It may be helpful to have a second bag in the car when away all day as a backup. This helps ensure if more supplies are used than usual, there is always an emergency bag of supplies available.

Remember, with an individual who requires supplies, it is not easy to go to a store and purchase it, so having the items on hand makes it more comfortable and easier on everyone. Also, a hospital may not carry the particular item. If they do have it, their pricing is generally much higher than you would normally pay. This is something to watch for if you have insurance limits to consider so you do not incur any undue out-of-pocket expenses.

In this section, you will notice that in some areas, there are two (2) forms: one a sample explaining the form for quick reference for any items needed when leaving the home and another for you to complete and customize to meet your needs.

You can contact Life Cycles Publishing office at info@LCPBooks.com to obtain a digital disc of forms that are included in the *Personal Caregiver Handbook* for you to customize to meet your individual needs. Please remember all forms are copyrighted protected.

Personal Bag Organization

Sample form for quick reference for any items needed when leaving the home.

*SUPPLIES CAN VARY DEPENDING ON THE PERSONAL NEEDS.

I. **Medications**

    A. **Pharmacy** _____ Phone _____

       Location _____

       ❑ Pickup ❑ Delivery option available ❑ Bubble pack (check with pharmacist) ❑ _____

       Type ❑ Rx ❑ Over the counter ❑ Other _____

    B. **Pharmacy** _____ Phone _____

       Location _____

       ❑ Pickup ❑ Delivery option available ❑ Bubble pack (check with pharmacist) ❑ _____

       Type ❑ Rx ❑ Over the counter ❑ Other _____

II. **Medical Supplier** – See Personal Supply list

    A. **Name** _____ **Phone** _____

       Delivery: ❑ Home delivery ❑ Pickup ❑ Auto ❑ Monthly ❑ Call frequency

       Type of supplies _____

    B. **Name** _____ **Phone** _____

       Delivery: ❑ Home delivery ❑ Pickup ❑ Auto ❑ Monthly ❑ Call frequency _____

       Type of supplies _____

III. **Various Bags/Case Supplies**

    A. **Backpack.** Attached to back of wheelchair or a side bag for a walker, paying close attention to balance, ensuring the weight of the bag does not cause instability.

       1. Daily check and restock to ensure that it contains all necessary items.

       2. All-day excursions may require more supplies. Some outings may require the following:

          a. Additional clothes in the event of an incontinence issue

          b. Personal supplies

          c. Additional cushion covers

          d. _____

    B. **Hip Bag/Purse.** Attached to wheelchair or walker

       1. This is the individual's responsibility; however, it may require the assistance of someone to ensure that they have what is needed.

2. For a female, it could be a purse; for a male, it could be just a wallet in a small pack with additional items.

   a. Wallet with some type of identification and medical card

   b. Other miscellaneous personal items

   c. Cell phone, emergency phone numbers, etc.

   d. Extra medication needed while away from home. This may be also carried in the backpack.

C. **Hospital Medical Supply Bag/Emergency Bag.** Always take the *Personal Medical Summary.* Located _____

   1. It is helpful to have a bag prepared for an emergency with all the daily personal supplies needed.

   2. Be sure to include any special medical supplies or personal items to ensure availability, and it can keep some of the hospital costs down.

      a. If a particular brand of diaper/brief is used, that may help reduce the incidence of a decubitus. The medical facility generally only has one type. You may want bring your own that fits properly and is more comfortable.

      b. If there are allergies to certain materials, such as *latex.* It is best to carry all latex-free items as not all hospitals or doctor offices have the same supplies.

      c. If there are ostomy supplies or catheters used, the size and product is individualized. Taking your own supplies ensures you have what is needed always.

      d. Always bring your *Personal Medical Summary, Personal Medical Journal,* pertinent X-rays, and any medical, surgical, and/or laboratory reports to assist the medical team.

D. **Travel Suitcase/Bag**
   Located _____.

   1. *Always* include current X-rays and *Personal Medical Summary* in case an emergency occurs.

   2. Pack depending on the current medical needs and supplies.

   3. Set out the clothes needed per day and include extra clothing and supplies should an incontinence event occur that will require additional changes.

   4. Keep in mind whether you will need to do laundry while away. This will alter the number of items you are packing.

E. **X-ray Case**

Located _____

1. Black zipper art case holds X-rays nicely. You can purchase a case at the local art supply store.

2. *Never, never, never* allow the X-rays to stay at the hospital unless the physician has personal custody, and they are being used for a procedure. This is personal history and critical for each physician to use in the different locations. They are critical to have when traveling in case of an emergency.

3. Take when you go to
    ✓Emergency
    ✓Hospital
    ✓Procedure being considered
    ✓If needed for a doctor appointment

F. **Grooming/Makeup Bag**

Located _____

1. Caregiver may handle or they may assist the individual.

2. List of items to consider

    Located _____

    1. _____
    2. _____
    3. _____
    4. _____
    5. _____
    6. _____
    7. _____
    8. _____
    9. _____
    10. _____

G. **Other** _____

    Located _____

    1. _____
    2. _____
    3. _____
    4. _____

5. _____

6. _____

7. _____

8. _____

9. _____

10. _____

Personal Bag Organization

Fill-in sample form for you to customize to meet your needs.

*SUPPLIES CAN VARY DEPENDING ON THE PERSONAL NEEDS.

I. **Medications**

    A. **Pharmacy** _____ Phone _____

        Location _____

        ❑ Pickup ❑ Delivery option available ❑ Bubble pack (check with pharmacist) ❑ _____

        Type ❑ Rx ❑ Over the counter ❑ Other _____

    B. **Pharmacy** _____ Phone _____

        Location _____

        ❑ Pickup ❑ Delivery option available ❑ Bubble pack (check with pharmacist) ❑ _____

        Type ❑ Rx ❑ Over the counter ❑ Other _____

II. **Medical Supplier.** See Personal Supply list.

    A. **Name** _____ Phone _____

        Delivery: ❑ Home delivery ❑ Pickup ❑ Auto ❑ Monthly ❑ Call frequency _____

        Type of supplies _____

    B. **Name** _____ Phone _____

        Delivery: ❑ Home delivery ❑ Pickup ❑ Auto ❑ Monthly ❑ Call frequency _____

        Type of supplies _____

III. **Bag and Case Supplies**

    A. **Backpack.** Attached to back of wheelchair or a side bag for a walker, paying close attention to balance and ensuring the weight of the bag does not cause instability.

        1. _____

        2. _____

        3. _____

        4. _____

    B. **Hip Bag or Purse.** Attached to wheelchair or walker.

        This is the individual's responsibility; however, it may require the assistance of someone to ensure that they have what is needed.

        1. _____

        2. _____

        3. _____

        4. _____

C. **Hospital Medical Supply Bag and Emergency Bag.** ❑ See attached list

Always take your *Personal Medical Summary.*

Located _____

1. It is helpful to have a bag prepared for an emergency with all the daily personal supplies needed.

2. Be sure to include any special medical supplies or personal items to ensure availability.

3. When you take your own personal daily supplies, it can help keep some of hospital costs down. Most hospitals charge more for various supplies you may use than you normally pay.

Make a list of what supplies you want to be included in your bag. You may need to add an additional sheet.

1. _____
2. _____
3. _____
4. _____
5. _____
6. _____
7. _____
8. _____

D. **Travel Suitcase and Bag.** ❑ See attached list.

Located _____

1. _____
2. _____
3. _____
4. _____
5. _____
6. _____
7. _____
8. _____

E. **X-ray Case**

Located _____

1. Black zipper art case holds X-rays nicely. You can purchase a case at the local art supply store.

2. *Never, never, never* allow the X-rays to stay at the hospital unless the physician has personal custody, and they are being used for a procedure. This is personal history and

critical for each physician to use in the different locations. They are critical to have when traveling in case of an emergency.

3. _____

4. _____

5. _____

6. _____

F. **Grooming and Makeup Bag**

Located _____

1. _____

2. _____

3. _____

4. _____

5. _____

6. _____

7. _____

8. _____

9. _____

10. _____

G. **Other**

Located _____

1. _____

2. _____

3. _____

4. _____

5. _____

6. _____

7. _____

8. _____

9. _____

10. _____

20
Personal Medical Summary

Using this form provides a medical history summary that should be shown to your physician at each visit and especially the emergency team so they can be sure of the medical history you have. The physicians today must move quickly between each patient that by providing your medical summary, it can assist them. Even if all the information is in the computer, this helps simplify and provide a quick resource of invaluable information that, if needed, you can refer to and remind them.

Physicians even in medical facilities that have everything computerized find this form extremely helpful and utilize it. It shows you care about your health, and they appreciate it.

When traveling, this offers you the information in the event you need to seek medical assistance.

It is important to summarize your past and current health information.
- If you are unable to recall the exact date, use the approximate year.
- Surgeries and procedures – If you do not remember the exact name, give a brief explanation.
- Complete as much history as you can remember and feel free to include all pertinent information that will be helpful during an emergency or medical treatment.
- Be sure to update as needed at least every six months to ensure the information is correct. Sometimes a medication is changed, and this way, you will have the current information.
- If you have an emergency and unable to speak for yourself, this will help the person assisting you to ensure the medical team has your up-to-date information.
- Make copies of your summary and keep a current master for your files. Take a picture of it and send it to your cell phone for a copy as well keep a copy in your book bag.

Personal Medical Summary

Keep this summary updated and present it to your medical/dental professional at *all* visits.

Name *(Last, First, M. I.)*			☐ M ☐ F	DOB	
Marital status	E-mail address				
Address		City		ST	Zip
Phone	Fax		Mobile	Work	
SS no. Xxx-xx-	Blood Type	Religion	Mother's maiden name		
Nearest relative		Phone	Relationship		

Medications Currently Taking

☐ See attached sheet for more information.

	Date	Drug	Dosage	Amount	Frequency	Purpose
1						
2						
3						
4						
5						
6						
7						
8						
9						
10						

Instructions

PURPOSE: To assist your medical/dental provider with your current up-to-date information for their files and to ensure that their information is current. Use as a condensed summary of your personal medical history.

Suggestions:

1. Before filling out forms, make extra copies to ensure availability of more forms to update as needed.

2. Be sure to take your *Personal Medical Summary* with you to all appointments that may need your medical history, including schools.

3. Take a copy with you when traveling to ensure you have the information you may need at your fingertips in the event you become ill or have an emergency.

Although the author has made every effort to ensure the accuracy and completeness of information contained in this form, she assumes no responsibility for errors, inaccuracies, omissions, or any inconsistency herein.

For more information or to order replacement forms, contact **Life Cycles Publishing, Inc.** at PO Box 41122, San Jose, CA 95160, www.lcpbooks.com or info@lcpbooks.com, (844)-527-2665.

Name _____

Allergies <u>Medications</u>

☐ See attached sheet for more information.

	Date	Medication	Reaction	Counterapplication (What did you take or do to relieve the allergy?)
1.				
2.				
3.				
4.				
5.				
6.				
7.				
8.				
9.				
10.				

➤ Note: Generic Rx products　　　* Yes　　　* No

Allergies <u>Foods</u>

	Date	Medication	Reaction	Counterapplication (What did you take or do to relieve the allergy?)
1.				
2.				
3.				
4.				
5.				
6.				
7.				
8.				
9.				
10.				

Name _____

Medical Conditions Diagnosis

☐ See attached sheet for more information.

	Date	Diagnosis	Problem	Comment
1.				
2.				
3.				
4.				
5.				
6.				
7.				
8.				
9.				
10.				

Alerts or Medical Illnesses

Health notation: Something you and/or your doctor/therapist are watching or monitoring.

☐ See attached sheet for more information.

	Date	Physician	Description	Concerns/Comment
1.				
2.				
3.				
4.				
5.				
6.				
7.				
8.				
9.				
10.				

Name _____

Surgeries/Hospitalizations

☐ See attached sheet for more information.

	Date	Hospital, City, State	Procedure	Comment
1.				
2.				
3.				
4.				
5.				
6.				
7.				
8.				
9.				
10.				

Tests, X-rays, Procedures

☐ See attached sheet for more information.

	Date	Hospital, City, State	Procedure	X-ray	Purpose	Results
1.						
2.						
3.						
4.						
5.						
6.						
7.						
8.						
9.						
10.						

Name _____

Family History

	Date	Diagnosis	Relative	Comment
1.				
2.				
3.				
4.				
5.				

➢ Please note important information that has not been stated.

_____

_____

_____

_____

_____

_____

_____

_____

Immunizations

Date	Physician	Immunization	Next Due	Purpose	Reactions
		Tetanus			
		Influenza			
		Pneumonia			
		MMR (measles-mumps-rubella)			

Name _____

Physicians, Dentist, Service Providers

	Date	Name	Address, City, State, Zip	Phone	Specialty

Insurance Information

Medical Provider/s _____ _____ _____
_____

Medical No. _____ Other Hospital No. _____ _____
_____

Medicare No. _____ Medi-Cal/State Provider No._____
Other _____
Subscriber _____ Subscriber No._____
Effective _____
Member Services Phone No. (___)_____ (___)_____
Deductible $ _____ Co Pay $ _____ Office Visit $ _____ Hospital $ _____
Emergency $ _____ Out of Service/Plan Area $ _____ Other $ _____
Medication: Generic $ _____ Non-Generic $ _____

Name _____

Primary Physician _____

Plan Code _____

Employer _____

Address _____

Phone ( ) _____

Dentist _____

Carrier _____ Plan Code_____

Address _____

Phone ( ) _____

Check with the doctor office or plan administrator regarding the fee schedule.

Other Coverage _____

Carrier _____ Plan Code_____

Check with the doctor office or plan administrator regarding the fee schedule.

Notes. ❑ See attached sheet.

_____

_____

_____

_____

_____

_____

_____

_____

_____

_____

_____

_____

_____

_____

_____

_____

_____

➤ Add a separate page for any notes you feel are important regarding your health that you want to ensure your medical/dental team are informed.

21
Personal Medical Supplies

It is important to have a list of all the supplies used and the reorder information. Always include the medical supplier contact information and how it is billed, either through your insurance, personal funding, or another source. By having this available, it makes it easier when you need to reorder. Also, note how it is sent to you, the type of mail service, and how the time it takes to receive your supplies once you have place the order.

Some suppliers have an auto reorder system. Be sure to communicate with them if you want them to automatically reorder the supplies and charge your bank account. You can discuss options that make it comfortable with you and your finances if you are paying for an item. You can request to have them call you prior to all orders to confirm if you need the product, and it will warn you the funds will be taken from your bank account on an agreed schedule.

It will be important to keep the list up to date so the correct supplies are ordered, and there is no delay when you need to rely on a particular item. It is important to remember that generally, when you order personal medical supplies, they do not have a return policy. It can be difficult to obtain a replacement order, and you may have to incur the additional financial cost.

Depending on how you order your supplies, it is helpful to have a form that the caregiver or the individual who requires the items can order from, especially if they need to fax it to the supplier. Be sure to check the information listed regarding the product, amount requesting, and the product number hasn't changed; and any new item that you are now using will need to be added.

When your supplies arrive, always check the invoice against your order form to ensure you have received everything you requested. Be sure to note if an item is on back order and call the supplier to find out when you will receive it.

Personal Medical Supplies

SUPPLIES CAN VARY DEPENDING ON PERSONAL NEEDS AT THE TIME

I.	**MEDICATIONS**	Attach the medication list from your Medical Provider, a copy from your Personal Medical Journal Medication Section, or make a list.
		Service Provider
		Phone

II.	**DAILY SUPPLIES**	Service Provider
		Phone

	Date Checked	# On Hand	Requires	Date Ordered	Monthly Order / Receives	On-Call / Phone In Only	Product Company	Order #	Product Description
1									
2									
3									
4									
5									
6									
7									
8									
9									
10									
11									
12									
13									
14									
15									
16									
17									
18									
19									
20									

22
Endorsement and Other Publications Available

ENDORSEMENT

Ms. Lopez would appreciate your endorsement. Please complete the attached endorsement sheet and return as stated on the form.

OTHER PUBLICATIONS AVAILABLE

A list of other publications is listed. Return the completed form for more information or additional copies.

Ms. Lopez is always available as a speaker at your organization or a meeting. Call to schedule a time to hear her and the wonderful wealth of information that she offers.

LIFE CYCLES PUBLISHING, INC.

P.O. Box 41122, San Jose, CA 95160 –www.lcpbooks.com – (844)527-2665

RE: ENDORSEMENT

As you are a valued individual, I would appreciate if you would consider providing me with your endorsement regarding the importance of maintaining your personal medical history to eliminate medical errors.

❑ All   ❑ Personal Medical Journal   ❑ My Personal Medical Journal   ❑ Personal Medical Pocket Journal

❑ Personal Care Handbook   ❑ Personal Caregiver Handbook

Please keep your comment brief preferably to one to three lines.

_____

_____

_____

How would you want your name to appear?

Name _____

Title _____

Business _____

Other _____

I give permission to use the above statement in:

❑All literature to include the following:

❑ Books - either on the front or back cover and not limited within the text content.

❑ Website - Internet

❑ Social Media   ❑ All   ❑ Except _____

❑ Newspapers, magazines, periodicals

❑ I would like to be kept informed when my name will be applied to anything.

❑ I want to limit this endorsement to the following: _____

_____

_____

Signed_____Date_____

Phone_____E-mail_____

Please either   Mail this to   Life Cycles Publishing   E-mail: Info@lcpbooks.com
P.O. Box 41122
San Jose, CA 95160

Should you have any questions, please do not hesitate to contact the office.

In appreciation,

Gloria Lopez, CEO/Author

LIFE CYCLES PUBLISHING, INC.

P.O. Box 41122, San Jose, CA 95160 – www.lcpbooks.com – (844)527-2665

Books available from Life Cycles Publishing, Inc. and Author Gloria Lopez for purchase

The following items are available for purchase individually and in bulk.

Consider giving this as a gift that will further aid your clients. Call us to find out more regarding customizing the cover to include your business name.

They can provide you or your clients the opportunity to maintain personal medical history, eliminating memorization and medical errors through documentation. It also provides the tools needed when working with various professionals.

❑ *Personal Medical Journal*   Spiral Bound 254-page self-help journal
   Maintains an individual's personal medical history from pregnancy and throughout their lifetime.

❑ *My Personal Medical Journal*   ❑ Hard Cover ❑ Soft Cover 230-page self-help journal
   Maintains an individual's personal medical history throughout their lifetime.

❑ *Personal Medical Pocket Journal*   3.5" X 7" 32-page self-help journal
   A condensed pocket summary of an individual's health history.
   Easy to carry in a purse or pocket.

❑ *Personal Care Handbook*   Soft Cover 144-page self-help handbook ❑ E-book ❑ Forms Disc
   Provides an individual with a chronic medical condition requiring the assistance of a caregiver to explain in detail their medical needs, disability, medical concerns, and all medical supplies needed and how to hire a caregiver.

❑ *Personal Caregiver Handbook* Soft Cover 158-page self-help handbook ❑ E-book ❑ Forms Disc
   Used daily by a caregiver with instructions and a variety of daily charting forms depending on the individual needs to assist in monitoring their health. The charts can be a helpful tool to take to the doctor appointment.

❑ Food Allergy Card

Used to present to waitresses and/or chefs to notify them of food allergies the person may have toward specific foods and spices.

✓ Eliminate potential cross-contamination, allowing the restaurant to prepare the food safely.

✓ Cards will be customized to include your company logo.

❑ I am interested in more information and the possibility of purchasing. Please check the above books of interest.

Name _____ Title _____

Company _____

Phone _____ E-mail _____